Yoga for Chronic Illness Bundle

Yoga for Chronic Pain, Yoga for Chronic Fatigue, and Yoga for Insomnia

Kayla Kurin

KAYLA KURIN

Yoga for Chronic Illness Bundle

www.arogayoga.com

© 2019 Kayla Kurin

info@arogayoga.com

Cover photography: Olivia Annand

YOGA FOR CHRONIC ILLNESS

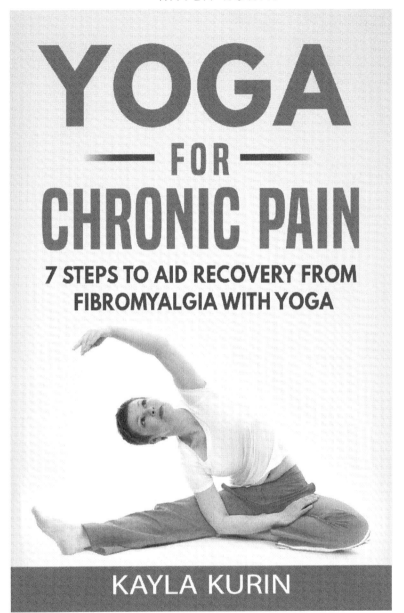

YOGA
— FOR —
CHRONIC PAIN
7 STEPS TO AID RECOVERY FROM FIBROMYALGIA WITH YOGA

KAYLA KURIN

Yoga for Chronic Pain

7 steps to aid recovery from fibromyalgia with yoga

Kayla Kurin

KAYLA KURIN

Yoga for Chronic Pain: 7 Steps to Aid Recovery From Fibromyalgia with Yoga by Kayla Kurin.

www.arogayoga.com

Cover photography: CC0 public domain
Book photography: Sarah Bouchard

Contents

Dear reader,

How are you feeling right now? On a scale of 1-10?

Can I guess that you are somewhere on the pain side of things? Can I also imagine that your pain isn't going away? Whether you take medication, go to what feels like hundreds of doctors appointments, go for walks in nature, or rest - the next day, you're still in pain. And how many times has someone promised you they could fix it if you have a few thousand dollars to fork over, but you've still come out feeling the same?

I wish I could reach out of the pages of this book and give you a great big hug because I know how it feels to be in terrible pain - for years, I woke up in pain and was exhausted all day. Even worse, no doctor could tell me how to fix it. I tried so many different things: different doctors, naturopaths, sleeping pills and supplements that tasted like dirt. Sometimes, the medication would work for a time, but mostly, it was just covering up the problem. I went on like this for years, feeling like I was only living half a life.

Despite some people thinking I was depressed or just lazy, I wanted to be doing the things my friends were doing. I wanted to be playing sports, attending classes, and travelling. But I couldn't do any of it, no matter what I tried.

After I had been living with illness for almost 7 years, someone recommended I try yoga. I said no. I didn't think it would work for me. My illness was serious; I wasn't a bit stressed out or looking for a new way to exercise. Then, another person recommended I try meditation. I also said no. If a doctor couldn't help me, I had no idea how a few breathing exercises would do anything. Instead, I continued bouncing between doctors and trying different medications. Finally, after my 7 year anniversary with the illness, I picked up a yoga DVD. It couldn't hurt, could it?

Ten years after picking up that yoga DVD, I'm still in recovery. After 2 years of a dedicated yoga and meditation practice (along with some other health and lifestyle changes I made), I stopped having regressions. I was able to do more and more with my day without worrying that I'd pay for it later. My pain lessened, and the fatigue began to lift.

Yoga and meditation led me to a new way of thinking about my body and about what the words 'illness' and 'health' mean.

It gave me the tools I needed to manage my pain and fatigue, and live a full life, even when I wasn't feeling my best. Eventually, it led to my full recovery.

I wondered why doctors weren't recommending yoga and meditation to patients with chronic fatigue and fibromyalgia. Was I an anomaly? So I started researching to see if I could find anyone else who had found recovery through yoga and if there was any science to back it up. The findings were astounding. The research was new, but it was showing that yoga and meditation were helpful for many chronic conditions and diseases. I found other stories of people who had found full or partial recovery through yoga, and over the 10 years since I've been practising, yoga is slowly making its way into mainstream medical advice.

As I began to prepare to write this book, the studies I found left me in awe of the power of the body-mind/mind-body connection. Western medicine is an incredible tool and has helped cure many illnesses that used to lead to death or disability. Yet, the way that western medicine breaks up the body into parts or diseases into symptoms often overlooks a big part of the way our bodies function. While this outlook can be helpful for acute illnesses, in the case of a chronic condition like Fibromyalgia, it's leaving a lot of people without proper treatment.

I don't think we need to do away with western medical practices. Eastern and western medicinal traditions complement each other, and we should use them together. Universal healing strategies like deep breathing, yoga, diet, etc. can be used in conjunction with specific healing strategies like the right medication or surgery. I prefer to use the word complementary medicine rather than alternative medicine because we don't need to choose one or the other. We should use all the tools we have to promote healing.

I mentioned that yoga and mindfulness didn't only change the way I felt, it changed my perspective on life. I realized that I wanted to live a life that helped others, and that was supportive of my health. It was for these reasons I decided to become a yoga teacher, and now, write this book.

I hope this book will help you to understand your pain better, and give you a variety of tools to manage your pain on your journey to recovery.

This book contains 7 steps that will help you understand your pain, and practical tips you can use to feel better. The first 2 steps focus on understanding your pain and cover both the scientific and yogic perspectives on pain management. These chapters help explain why yoga and meditation have been so helpful to so many people. If you're having a brain fog kind of day, you might not take everything in from these chapters, but that's okay. The next 5 steps focus on practical things you can try, and they are the most crucial part of the book. As Pattabhi Jois, the found of Ashtanga yoga, says:

"Yoga is 1% theory and 99% practice"

If you'd like to skip straight to a yoga practice, feel free to head over to the **'free videos'** page on my website (www.arogayoga.com), and get started with a short home yoga practice.

If you're ready to get started with a deeper understanding of yoga and mindfulness, then happy reading!

Sending light and love,

Kayla

Step 1: Understanding Your Pain

Pain is a neural signal from your body to your brain (and sometimes from your brain to your body!) telling you that something is wrong. Pain can be acute or chronic and can feel sharp, dull, throbbing, or ever-present. It can be a small amount of pain like a dull ache, or it can be debilitating pain that keeps you from participating in or enjoying your daily life.

Acute pain is short-lived, and usually a sign you've injured yourself in some way. For example, stubbing your toe or breaking an arm. Chronic pain is more complex and can have a variety of causes. Chronic pain can be in one or several areas of the body, but it's most common in the joints, lower back, shoulders, neck, and head. Sometimes, illness or lifestyle choices (e.g. Bad posture) can cause pain. However, pain does not always have a known cause.

Chronic pain can be something present all the time such as in Arthritis and Fibromyalgia. It can also be intermittent but constant such as migraine headaches.

While feeling pain can be worrisome, it isn't necessarily harmful. It is your body's way of communicating with the brain and pain can be there to protect you from further injuring yourself, or letting a severe illness go untreated. Of course, feeling pain all the time when you don't know the cause can be very stressful.

We used to have a simplistic understanding of pain - that it signalled the brain as a direct result of a physical stimulus. Yet, further research on pain is proving that this is not always in true. In many cases, there is no physical damage present, but the patient can still be experiencing intense pain.

Pain, no matter the cause, makes your 'fight or flight' reaction go off. When the pain is acute, this can be a helpful reaction. If you've been attacked and feel pain, you know it's time to run away. If you've put your hand too close to a burning flame, you know not to do it again.

However, when it comes to chronic pain, if your fight or flight (known as the sympathetic nervous system) is always on high alert, this can cause you more pain and make it harder to heal.

The fight or flight response is part of the autonomic nervous system (ANS). Within the ANS there's the sympathetic (fight or flight) system and the parasympathetic (rest and digest) system.

The fight or flight response is a normal healthy response to some situations. If there's a bear in the room, we want our sympathetic nervous system to activate. Yet, it becomes a dysfunction when it turns on for fibromyalgia pain that is constant, instead of giving the body a chance to rest and heal.

When the sympathetic nervous system is activated, you'll notice that:

- Your heart rate increases

- Your muscles tense

- Digestion slows down

- Your breath becomes shallow

- Your palms begin to sweat

If you've ever gotten butterflies in your stomach before doing something you were nervous about, you've experienced the effects of the sympathetic nervous system. If you're living with fibromyalgia, you may even feel as though you experience those things on a daily basis.

When the parasympathetic nervous system is activated, you'll notice that:

- Digestions improves

- Your muscles relax

- Your heart rate slows down

- You can breathe deeper

Which one of these symptoms would you guess promotes better healing for chronic pain? I think we can all agree it's the second one. The parasympathetic nervous system creates the space that the body needs to heal and relax. Treating the symptoms of pain by taking painkillers or getting a massage won't have any lasting effect if we can't learn to activate the parasympathetic nervous system and keep our muscles relaxed after the effects of the medication or treatment wear off.

The yogic view on suffering is somewhat different than the traditional scientific view of pain. However, recent research on pain is starting to line up closer to the yogic idea of a mind-body connection.

As we said, pain is the way your body communicates danger to your brain. Yet, this danger may not always be a physical sensation, even if your brain perceives it that way. Let's take a look at an example:

Your child is playing outside, and trips on the curb, scraping her knee on the pavement. She starts to cry, and runs inside for you to 'fix it'. A few days later, your child is playing outside on the grass. She trips and falls, but this time she is met by soft ground rather than the pavement. What does your child do? She may get up and continue playing. She may begin crying again, even if there is no scrape this time. What you'll notice is, she'll pause for a moment. She knows what's supposed to happen when you fall over. It's supposed to hurt. This may cause her to start crying, thinking she's hurt. Or it may cause her to take a moment to register a new experience - it doesn't hurt to fall on the grass. If she does begin crying, does that mean she's a crybaby and not experiencing any real pain? Of course not. We already know that pain is viewed as signals the body sends to the brain. But it can sometimes work the other way around too. If your child's brain thinks falling is supposed to hurt, it may send pain signals to the body even if there is no physical damage.

Pain is not as straightforward as we once imagined. The way your body experiences pain depends on your expectations, experiences, and emotions at the time. It can depend on whether help (mom) is nearby or not. It only takes a moment for your brain to process all these things, so it is a process not many of us are aware of. Once your brain has processed this information, it will decide on how high the sensation of pain should be. Ie. It will tell your conscious brain how much danger it thinks you're in.

In the yogic world, the mind and body are irrevocably connected. If you find this model of pain trickier to understand, let's look at another example, going back to our 'fight or flight' response:

Let's say you're being chased in the woods by a wolf. As you're running, you trip and scrape your knee. In fact, you've tripped on the exact same root you did last week when you went for a run in the woods. That time, you went back to home to patch it up because it was too painful to continue running. However, this time, your brain decides that this pain is not as great as the pain that awaits you if you stop running. You probably won't feel any pain in your knee until your brain is convinced you are out of immediate danger. Once that happens, your brain will start to want you to pay attention to more minor threats, like a scraped or bruised knee.

This is an example to show you that pain is not always consistent. Even when living with chronic pain, the pain may ebb and flow depending on what else is going on in your life. It may depend on how well you slept last night, the weather, work or life stress, etc.

Many sufferers of fibromyalgia will be left without help because their doctors can't find a physical cause to their pain. However, the pain they're feeling in their bodies is genuine, despite lack of physical evidence for it. I remember when I studied psychology in university, we learned about amputees who can still feel sensation in limbs they've had amputated[i]. Up to 80% of amputees feel sensations in a limb that is no longer there, and most of these sensations are pain. This shows how little we know about how the body experiences pain. If you're living with fibromyalgia, you may be frustrated if people think you're 'faking it' or 'exaggerating' because no one can find a physical cause for your pain. Yet, if we look at pain research, this is not something unique to fibromyalgia. There have been several theories of what causes phantom limb pain, but scientists still aren't sure exactly what causes the pain.

Another example of how pain is not always physical is called sympathetic pain[ii]. Up to 25% of people experience sympathetic pain, which is the term applied to people who experience pain by seeing others in pain. This is especially true for parents who see their children in pain. Yet, even people watching the news or hearing stories of violence can experience sympathetic pain. I mention these theories to show that just because you are experiencing an intense physical sensation of pain, it doesn't mean the cause is physical. It can be a combination of a number of things that are a part of your environment. It in no way implies that the pain you're experiencing isn't a real, physical sensation.

Understanding that you may be able to treat pain not by treating a physical cause, but by addressing the environment that creates the pain (such as stress, thought patterns, sleeping habits, beliefs, etc.) is a massive breakthrough in the world of pain research. More than that, it starts to explain why so many people find yoga, meditation, and mindfulness a useful tool for managing chronic pain. Yoga sees the body and mind as connected. It's a two-way street.

The western world often takes a specific approach to pain. Rather than looking at the whole person and trying to create balance, it tries to pinpoint the pain and either remove the cause or dull the symptoms. This approach can be beneficial in cases of acute pain. If you break your arm, you should go to the doctor and have the specific symptom (broken arm) treated. No matter how much yoga or meditation you do, you won't stop the pain until you've fixed the cause of the pain.

But sometimes this approach isn't so practical. I remember once I was advised to 'not run if I felt knee pain when running'. A holistic approach would be to refer me to a physiotherapist who might be able to correct my running stride or a muscular imbalance in my legs. It also went wrong for me when I went from sleeping pill to sleeping pill to sleeping pill, desperate to find a good night's sleep. But the pills weren't helping me get to the root of the problem, which was hyper-arousal before bed. They can provide a temporary fix by forcing me to relax. But as soon as I built up a tolerance for the medication, there was my insomnia again. It wasn't until I learned how to deeply relax that I was able to sleep through the night.

Western medicine isn't equipped to deal with non-life threatening chronic conditions. Things like chronic pain or fatigue or insomnia are complicated issues. They don't often get priority in medical research because they aren't causing imminent danger.

This is why many people with chronic illnesses seek complementary medicine.

All that said, the scientific world is starting to take an interest in yoga and meditation. They've heard the stories of people like me who have used it to recover from illness, and are starting to study it. Research in the field is new but looks very promising. Many doctors are already beginning to recommend meditation or yoga to their patients living with chronic illnesses.

Action Steps

1) Start a journal or spreadsheet to track your progress over the next 2 months. Make a column to measure your pain levels, and start recording times you feel in pain. What happened the night before you had a pain flare? What happened an hour before? How long did it last?

Step 2: Understanding The Science of Yoga

Yoga is more than just a form of exercise. It comes from a medical system called Ayurveda, which is over 2000 years old and originates in ancient India. Ayurveda is often referred to as yoga's sister science and is still practised in India and other places around the world. In India, some Ayurvedic doctors and hospitals have adapted ancient systems to modern times.

Ayurveda takes a holistic approach to healthcare. Rather than treating symptoms, Ayurveda looks at the whole person.

It investigates your genetic makeup and emotional patterns, and how this affects your health. This is why, when we look at how yoga can help you manage or recover from fibromyalgia (or any illness) we don't look just at the yoga postures. We also look at your mind, body, breath, and lifestyle.

I found Ayurveda helpful in my recovery process because treating the symptoms (which is what my doctor was recommending) wasn't helping me. Without getting to the root cause of the issue, I was only getting Band-Aid solutions.

My doctors were confused about what chronic fatigue and fibromyalgia were. It's hard to cure something you don't understand. Because Ayurvedic medicine takes a holistic approach to healthcare, they can identify the combination of things (such as genetics, bacterial imbalances, emotional blockages or thought patterns, physical ailments, or lifestyle choices) that may be causing your illness.

Another reason why I love the Ayurvedic approach to healthcare is that it doesn't put everyone in the same category. In Ayurveda, there are three main doshas, or dispositions, that we each have. Most people will be dominant in one or two of these doshas, but, some people are balanced between all three. When one of the doshas is out of balance, it can cause mild or temporary symptoms, but if the dosha goes unbalanced for too long, it can lead to serious illness.

If you visit an Ayurvedic doctor, the first thing that they'll do is determine your dosha. Instead of looking only at your symptoms, they'll look at your body type, emotional patterns, and genetic dispositions to determine which kinds of viruses, events, or lifestyle choices may trigger illness in you. This can vary from person to person. For example, I now know that changing my diet (by removing gluten, dairy, and anything breaded or deep fried) made me feel a lot better. But a lot of my friends eat grilled cheese sandwiches and fish and chips and feel fine. It doesn't mean that there's anything wrong with me, it just means we have different dispositions that react differently to the same stimuli.

The three doshas are:

• Kapha: Content and deliberate, Kaphas have a broad, sturdy build, thick hair, smooth skin, and tend to move slowly. Kapha's will be drawn to slow types of movement like yin yoga and enjoy nurturing those around them.

- Pitta: Fiery and intense, Pitta's are quick to anger, and often have a medium build with yellowish or reddish skin and are prone to red hair and freckles. Pitta's are competitive and will be drawn to an active yoga practice like Ashtanga.

- Vata: Airy and scattered, Vata's love talking about many ideas and can never seem to get warm. They have a thin build often with knobbly joints. Vata's resist forming a routine, and are drawn to quick movements like a vinyasa class.

Ayurvedic principles hold that when one dosha is out of balance (whatever balance may mean for an individual's constitution), the imbalance can negatively affect the mind or body. If left untreated this can lead to illness. For example, when vata is out of balance, it can cause insomnia, anxiety, running thoughts, dry skin and nails, gas, bloating, brain fog, and a dislike of cold. To many with fibromyalgia, these symptoms will sound all too familiar. Insomnia, problems with memory, and trouble with digestion are all characteristic of fibromyalgia in addition to the pain.

Many things can cause vata to become imbalanced, such as

eating foods that are hard for you to digest, lifestyle choices, and psychological issues. If you are primarily a vata person, any stress can cause the dosha to become imbalanced. Also, keep in mind that stress weakens your immune system. If you went through a stressful period in life, this makes you more susceptible to picking up a virus, which could, in turn, lead to a dosha imbalance and a more severe illness like fibromyalgia.

In Ayurvedic medicine, there is no one size fits all cure. What is recommended to you by an ayurvedic practitioner will depend on your individual constitution. This is why in yoga, especially when practising yoga from a book or DVD; your body is always your best teacher. If any of the exercises later in this book make you feel worse, please stop immediately, and consult with your healthcare practitioner and a qualified yoga therapist before trying it again.

To balance the vata dosha, Ayurvedic medicine makes a few key recommendations:

1. Meditate to calm the mind

2. Use breath work to observe the energy in your body

3. Practice grounding asana postures to soothe the body

4. Reconsider your diet

5. Improve your sleep

6. Practice self-care for your mind, body, and soul

In the rest of this book, we'll get into detail with practical tips on how you can do these things. We'll also pull from scientific research to discover where it agrees with Ayurvedic principles and where it does not.

As you move through this book, remember that Ayurveda is an individualistic way of looking at medical treatment. Everything that works for me might not work for you and visa versa. However, we can look at best practices, and draw from what has worked for others. I can't promise you specific results, but I can tell you what has worked for me, and for my students to help us lead full and pain-free lives. I urge you to work your way through this book with an open mind, before deciding if it works or doesn't work for you. Once you've completed the book and given yourself 8 weeks to try out these steps, then you can decide which things you want to keep doing (if any) and which you want to drop.

I'm excited to embark on this healing journey with you as

we move on to the next step, taming the mind...

Action Steps

1) **Take this quiz** to find out what your dosha is. Then take **this quiz** to find out which doshas are out of balance. Remember to keep an open mind to the end of this book. See if there is anything helpful for you in understanding your dosha. If you're reading the print version of this book, head to yogainternational.com and search for 'dosha quiz' and then 'vikriti test'.

Step 3: Taming the Mind

In my 5 years as a yoga therapist, I cannot count how many people have told me they can't meditate or do yoga because they have a 'running mind'. If you also feel this way, you're not alone. The idea that we should 'turn off our minds' or 'stop thinking' during a yoga or meditation session is one of the most frustrating myths I come up against as a yoga therapist.

There's no way we can force our minds to stop thinking. Even when we sleep, we can't shut off our brains.

The goal of mindfulness is not to turn off your thoughts. The goal is to observe your thoughts as if from a distance. This objective stops you from getting emotionally involved with each idea as it enters your mind. After all, your thoughts are not facts. They're not the truth. They're just thoughts. When we become too invested in our thoughts, just like becoming too invested in your best friend's relationship drama, it can cause a drain on your energy levels and cause your stress levels to rise. The goal of mindfulness is to keep our stress levels manageable by interacting with our thoughts objectively.

Being mindful means, we are not worrying about the future or dwelling on the past. We might be observing thoughts or anxieties about those things, but our consciousness always stays in the present.

When we can observe our thoughts, we can also expand that awareness to other sensations and events around us. We become present in conversations with loved ones. We notice the sounds of nature or cars zooming past when out for a walk. We Notice the flavours in a dish a loved one has prepared. Or we enjoy the smell of freshly baked bread while passing by a bakery.

In mindfulness practice, we withhold judgement on the

sensations we are noticing. Our thoughts, the flavours of food, or the smells we're absorbing (even if it's the smell of a diaper that needs to be changed) don't need to be good or bad. We can simply observe their elements without judgement.

Mindfulness doesn't involve trying to change anything. And it certainly doesn't include trying to stop your thoughts. It just means that we are observing what is happening to and around us. Rather than becoming involved in every thought or sensation we experience.

What does the science say about mindfulness?

Thanks to John Kabat Zinn, the physician who is credited with bringing mindfulness to the western world, the effects on mindfulness meditation on health have been studied more than any other kind of complementary health practice.

In a meta-review (a type of scientific study which reviews a large body of studies done on a subject) done in 2017, it showed that mindfulness did help to decrease pain in chronic pain patients. Specifically symptoms of depression and low quality of life that often go with chronic pain.[iii]

Studies have also found that yoga has a more positive effect on health than other forms of exercise such as walking.[iv] Doctors have long known that exercise has a positive effect on mood and health. But why does yoga seem to have a stronger effect than other forms of exercise? We don't know for sure, but many in the yoga community believe that it is due to the mindfulness, meditation, and breath work that is used in a yoga practice, as well as the physical postures.

Despite mindfulness being the most researched area in complementary medicine, there is still a long way to go in discovering how mindfulness helps chronic pain sufferers. Due to the variant nature of pain and difficulty in measuring pain consistently from person to person, it can be a hard topic to study. However, many doctors are now recommending meditation to patients who don't respond to traditional treatments.

When it comes to mindfulness, one of the greatest benefits is that there is no harm in trying. While some people I've worked with are hesitant to try yoga because they don't want to make their symptoms worse by over-doing it with physical exercise or moving the wrong way, mindfulness doesn't come with any physical risk. You can practice mindfulness on your own, by listening to a recorded meditation track, or by working with a teacher trained in mindfulness meditation.

Primary and Secondary Suffering

Understanding the difference between primary and secondary suffering is essential to understanding how mindfulness can reduce chronic pain.

Primary suffering is the initial pain you experience after physical or emotional trauma. If you stub your toe, for example, that first shot of pain would be primary suffering.

For the most part, we can't help the way primary pain feels. It's caused by something external, and our reaction to it is out of our control, dictated by the subconscious systems of the body.

Secondary suffering is the pain we experience on top of the

initial shock. For example, if after stubbing your toe you think to yourself, 'Shit! This is the most painful thing that's ever happened to me! I'm sure it's broken!' That is secondary suffering. Most people won't jump to the conclusion that stubbing their toe means it's broken. Yet, when it comes to more serious conditions like relentless chronic pain, it's easy to fall into negative thought patterns. While thoughts like 'this pain will never go away', may seem realistic, they can actually make the pain worse.

We now know that the environment we're in (or help create) can affect the amount of pain we feel. So it makes sense that these negative thoughts can make your pain worse without any intention to do so on your part.

An initial adverse reaction to extreme or chronic pain is normal. In many situations, it's helpful. It helps your brain process not to do that harmful thing again (i.e. Walking without looking where you're going). However, when we don't know the cause of the pain, sustaining these negative thoughts are not helpful.

Stopping these negative thought patterns is easy to talk

about, but in practice, it's challenging.

Mindfulness is a tool that we can use to help 'reprogram' the brain and change these thought patterns. In mindfulness, we take a non-judgemental approach to our experiences. This non-judgement helps us differentiate from the pain our mind may be trying to tell us is present (I have fibromyalgia, I always feel pain) vs. the pain we are actually experiencing which can change from day to day and moment to moment.

When it comes to using mindfulness to reduce pain, we want to focus on the things we can control. We can choose to practice yoga or meditation; we can decide to monitor our breath; we can take a moment to notice sensations in our body.

Focusing on the things we can control also helps us set up for goals that we can achieve. For example, the goal to lose 10 pounds would not be an effective yogic goal. You can't control whether you'll be able to lose the weight. However, setting a goal to eat 7 servings of fruits and vegetables per day, or exercise 3 times per week, are both goals in which we can, for the most part, control the results.

Let's apply this principle to setting goals or expectations for chronic pain. Instead of thinking I want to try this new program, diet, doctor, etc. and be completely pain-free, you can set a goal to reduce the number of negative thought patterns or other lifestyle habits that may be contributing to your pain. It doesn't mean you'll be pain-free, but it does mean that you're taking steps to reduce your pain in a way that you can control.

To summarise, secondary pain is the pain that is most affected by us, by our thoughts, feelings, emotions, or lifestyle habits. It's the pain that we can control, and focus on reducing. The primary pain will still be present, but we can reduce the amount of pain we feel by lowering our secondary suffering.

Pain Acceptance

True, deep acceptance opens the path to healing. By accepting the pain present in our body, we can begin to reduce secondary suffering. If you start to become aware of pain at different points throughout the day, you'll begin to see that your pain is not constant. It may feel different at certain times of the day or when you're under stress vs. feeling relaxed. If you pay attention you'll realize your pain is not permanent - it is flowing and ever-changing. While this means your pain could get much worse, it also means your pain can get better. We don't know what will happen, all we do know is that the pain changes. As Heraclitus says: *"The only thing that is constant, is change".*

Thoughts like you'll never get better, that the pain will never go away, or that you'll never be able to do some of the things you had planned for your life, can all seem like realistic ways to grieve - and are all perfectly understandable thoughts to have. But, these thought patterns can add to your suffering. You don't know if your pain will go away or not. You don't know if it will get better or worse. All you know is what is happening in your body at the moment. We can't possibly know the outcome in the future, we can only try to accept the present.

When in pain, it's a normal response to want to fight and resist this pain. Phrases like "we can beat this" are common amongst patient groups and charities for illnesses. It feels like we're going to a championship sports match and want to win, not working with our bodies, which we love and cherish. What if the fighting approach, while a natural response, is the wrong way approach. What if this response is actually creating more pain rather than eliminating it?

What if instead of "I will beat this pain" we say "I will work with this pain and my body in a respectful way to live my fullest life."

Acceptance of your pain is not resignation. It is simply acknowledging the situation as it is in this moment. It is allowing yourself to stop struggling against yourself and letting peace and kindness take its place. Once you can make this transition, your stress levels, and secondary suffering will begin to diminish.

Stress and Pain

Stress makes all pain worse. It's also true that stress exacerbates any illness from the common cold to cancer. The bottom line is: stress is bad for your health. Once you start to become more aware of the flow of your pain, you'll be able to monitor better which activities are stressful and cause your pain to get worse or flare.

Stress combined with pain can create a cycle that is hard to break without mindful intention. You feel pain, which makes you feel stressed out, which makes you feel more pain, which makes you feel even more stressed out!

So how can you break this cycle?

We already know that pain is a signal that your body is giving you that something is wrong. This signal activates that sympathetic nervous system, or fight or flight response. If your pain is acute, or life-threatening, this response is necessary for survival. Your heart rate will increase, your breath will become shallow, your muscles will tense, your pupils will dilate, your palms might sweat, and that feeling of butterflies in your stomach? That's the muscles in your intestines slowing down movement. Your body is programming you to put all of your mental and physical energy towards stopping the threatening situation. When you're living with chronic pain, this response is exhausting.

Yoga and meditation systemically work to deepen your breath and relax your muscles. Researchers have found that yoga and meditation significantly lower levels of cortisol in the brain - cortisol is the hormone that is associated with stress.

Doing yoga or meditating can have a long-term effect on how we manage stress. Another study found that people who regularly meditate, bounce back from stress faster than those who do not regularly meditate[v]. What does this mean exactly? Let's take a look at this example:

You're out for a walk and want to cross the street. You're having a flare with severe brain fog and accidentally look the wrong way. You hear a car horn and jump out of the way just in time to avoid getting hit by a car. What's happening inside your body at this moment? The stress response is in full swing. Since this was a life-threatening situation, your body is appropriately responding to the situation. Those who don't meditate may carry the stress of that incident with them around for the rest of the day. But, those who regularly meditate or practice mindfulness can calm their bodies' down faster and return to normal levels of stress hormones after the upsetting incident.

Just as mindfulness doesn't mean stopping your thoughts, meditating or mindfulness doesn't mean you will always be calm and relaxed and never feels stressed. I feel stressed out all the time! However, if you build a regular mindfulness practice, you'll be able to better manage and overcome that stress. This means stress will be less of a drain on your energy sources that could be used for healing. At the very least, reducing stress won't make anything worse.

Not only can the pain itself be stressful, but thinking about pain or triggers for the pain can cause stress. For example, if you often have pain when you wake up in the morning, or after going for a walk, the anticipation and monitoring of that pain can cause even more stress. Being mindful helps us live in the moment, and let go of 'anticipation stress'.

Engaging in activities that help reduce stress on a regular basis such as yoga, meditation and systemic relaxation can all help reduce the amount of pain you experience. It's not just yoga and mindfulness that can help reduce stress. Partaking in a hobby you love, reading your favourite book, spending time outside, exercising, spending time with friends and family, and cooking your favourite meal can all help lower your stress levels.

Not all activities that we see as relaxing are actually relaxing. For example, spending a lot of time in front of a screen, especially at night time, can be arousing for the body. Watching movies or TV shows or reading books with a lot of violence or suspense can also stimulate the nervous system and make it hard to sleep.

If you have trouble sleeping, this is also something that can exacerbate pain. While we can't control whether we sleep, we can work to create the conditions for a good night's sleep by creating good sleep habits (more on this in chapter 6). We can also build a yoga practice designed to help rest. We'll go over what this could look like in the yoga chapter.

Mindfulness Practices

Mindfulness meditation focuses on building awareness. This may be awareness of the body, awareness of your thoughts, awareness of the senses, etc.

Some of the most popular types of mindfulness meditation are:

A Body Scan

A body scan involves moving your attention through different parts of your body and noticing feelings or sensations in your body. An important part of the body scan is to suspend judgement over whether these feelings are 'good' or 'bad'. You should just to notice how they feel. For example, is the feeling heavy or light? Tight or loose? Dull or aching? etc.

How to do it:

- Lie down on a yoga mat or your bed. Begin by focusing on your breath, breathing slowly and deeply.
- As you inhale, bring your focus down to your feet, noticing any sensations in your toes, heels, or the top or bottom of the feet. Hold your

attention here for 2-3 breaths. On the next exhale, release your attention.

- On the next inhale, move the attention up to the ankles and calves.

- Continue moving your attention through the body from your toes to your head, moving your focus every few breaths.

- Suspend passing judgement on the things you notice in your body. Allow any feelings to reside in your body - just for the moment.

- Finish the meditation by bringing your awareness to your entire body at once, and then slowly moving the fingers and the toes before sitting up.

Breathing Meditation

As you can guess from the name, this meditation focuses on your breath. You can visualize your breath moving in and out of the body and through the respiratory system; you can focus on physical sensations of the breathing; or count your breath to stay focused.

How to do it:

- Lie down or sit in a comfortable position free from distractions or interruptions.

- Begin by focusing on your breath. Notice how the breath feels moving in and out of your nostrils, all the way down into your diaphragm.

- Picture the breath moving into your nose, through your throat, through your lungs, and down into your belly. Imagine you can see the breath re-tracing this route back out into the room.

- After 5-10 rounds of visualizing your breath, count your breaths up to 10, then back down to 1, counting each breath on the exhale.

- Once you've come back to 1, take a few more breaths, noticing how your body feels, and then open your eyes.

Thought Observation

I mentioned earlier in this chapter that one of the pillars of mindfulness is observing your thoughts. This meditation helps you to actively observe your thoughts without becoming attached to them. This meditation can help reduce anxiety or overthinking. Thoughts are not facts or morsels of truth. They simply come and go as we inhale and exhale.

How to do it:

- Sit in a comfortable position free from distractions or interruptions, and start with a short breathing meditation.

- Slowly begin to shift your focus from your breath to your thoughts.

- Acknowledge the thoughts running through your mind and allow them to stay there, while still being aware of your breath, and what is happening in the present moment. I sometimes find it helpful to repeat my thoughts in my head by saying 'I'm thinking about what I want for dinner now, okay. I'm thinking about that really embarrassing moment where I fell in front of my co-workers earlier today okay that's fine, but right now I'm doing a meditation and am breathing, and am sitting, and am noticing.' , Etc.

- If you find yourself responding emotionally to your thoughts, or you spiral into a thought train, it can help to listen to a guided meditation so you have someone to remind you to come back to the present. This can be a difficult meditation, especially for those of us with 'monkey brain', but it can also be one of the most rewarding in reducing stress and anxiety.

- After 10-15 minutes bring your focus back to your breath to come out of the meditation.

Expanding Awareness

This meditation includes elements of the above three meditations. You begin this meditation by focusing on your breath. You can then extend that awareness to focus on the body. From there expand your awareness to the thoughts in your mind. Continue to expand your awareness to the sensations you feel on the skin, and the sound you feel around you. This is an advanced type of mindfulness meditation and you can continue until you have full awareness of yourself and the space around you.

How to do it:

- Sit in a comfortable position free from distractions.
- Start with a breathing meditation
- Move into a body scan meditation
- Move into a thought observation meditation

- Begin to bring your senses into awareness. What can you hear? Feel? Smell?
- Bring any other people or pets in the area into your awareness
- See if you can hold all of these things, both inside of you and outside of you in your awareness at once.
- Return to focusing on your breath or a breathing meditation
- Finish the meditation with a few slow breaths, and open your eyes.

Moving Meditation

When yoga originated, the physical postures were created to help monks stay physically healthy while sitting in meditation for long periods of time. One of my first yoga teachers told me that yoga was a moving meditation, and I've always kept that thought with me when I'm doing my physical yoga practice. However, a moving meditation isn't limited to yoga. It can be other forms of exercise like tai chi, chi gong, or even going for a slow walk while noticing how your body feels and your surroundings.

How to do it:

- Choose which activity you'd like to do mindfully. If it's yoga, you can follow some of the sequences later in this book, so for the purposes of this chapter, we'll cover a walking meditation.

- Find a place to walk or move that isn't too busy. You can do this inside your house, in a park, or on a quiet street. It's hard to stay focused in a meditation if you have to keep looking out for people or cars!

- Begin by standing, and doing a mini expanding meditation, first by focusing on your breath, and then your body.

- As you start to walk, notice how your body feels when moving. Notice how it feels on your feet to make contact with the ground with your feet. Notice which muscles you're using and how your body moves.

- If you find your mind starts to wander, it can be helpful to count your steps.

- Do this meditation for as long as you find it comfortable.

If you're new to meditation, I recommend starting with the body scan and breathing meditation. As you get more comfortable you can move onto the thought observation and expanding awareness meditations. Moving meditation is something that you can practice every day, either during your yoga practice, walking around your house, or going out for a walk in nature. We'll talk more about incorporating mindfulness into your daily life in the last chapter of this book.

Action Steps

1) Set a mindful goal for your pain management plan. What can you commit to doing where you will have control over the results? Write this goal down and stick it up somewhere in your house where you will see it every day. Also add this goal to your tracking sheet from step 1.

2) Choose one of the mindfulness practices mentioned in this chapter and practice it for 10 minutes, 3 times this week. Record how you feel before and after in a journal.

Step 4: Using the Breath as an Energy Source

While mindfulness focuses on observing and giving attention to the breath, pranayama focuses on controlling the breath.

Pranayama is the Yogic word for breath control or breathing exercises. Prana is the Sanskrit word for breath or life force. Ayama means to restrain or control. These exercises are intended to clear any blocks you have so that the prana can flow freely through you. The concept of prana is similar to the idea of chi in traditional Chinese medicine.

If you go to a yoga class in a gym or a yoga studio focused on fitness, the amount of meditation and breathing exercises in the class may be limited. However, if you are working with a yoga therapist, meditation and breath work will become an essential part of your yoga practice.

One thing I love about breath work and meditation in the treatment of chronic pain is that, just like mindful meditation, you can do them every day. Even on days when you feel in too much pain or too tired to do a physical yoga practice (or get out of bed), you can still do a breathing exercise.

In the body, we have voluntary and involuntary actions. Voluntary actions are things we do consciously, such as walking, talking, eating, etc. Involuntary actions are things that happen automatically such as your heart beating, digestion of food, etc. Breathing is an involuntary activity - if you try to stop breathing, you'll pass out, and your body will automatically start breathing for you again. Yet, we can also control our breath to some extent. We can hold our breath, breathe deeply, breathe shallowly, through the nose, through the mouth, noisily, quietly, etc. It's because of this reason that yogi's see pranayama as an essential daily routine. It connects both the voluntary and involuntary systems.

Because breathing is the only involuntary system we can control, breathing practices can be a powerful tool to 'uncouple' other automatic associations we make. For example, your negative emotions or pain can become part of your identity. Sometimes, we subconsciously hold on to suffering because we see it as a part of who we are. You may also associate certain triggers or actions with pain, and breaking these associations can help reduce pain. You can't completely break these associations, but we can reduce it, so you don't feel as overwhelmed by the pain.

When I started practising yoga, I only practised mindfulness meditations. As I learned more about pranayama, I began incorporating these breathing exercises into my daily practice. I used to have a chronically stuffed nose and struggled to breathe through it. When I started practising some of the yogic breathing exercises below, my sinuses cleared up, and for the first time that I could remember, I was able to breathe through my nose!

I recommend practising both pranayama and mindfulness or other forms of meditation. Pranayama can help prepare the mind for meditation and can help you get into a deeper meditative state - thus increasing the health benefits of meditation.

Breathing is a thing we do all day, every day. But it can be a powerful tool for improving your health by paying attention to it or controlling it. Diaphragmatic breathing (breathing deeply into your diaphragm, so your belly rises on each inhalation) is refreshing and restful and creates a sense of well-being. It calms the nervous system, helps prevent psychosomatic disturbances, including panic episodes, and centres attention. Because we are always breathing, breath awareness is a self-management tool that is useful even during the busiest times of the day.

Here are some of my favourite pranayama exercises:

Alternate nostril breathing

☐

While alternate nostril breathing was recently made famous by Hilary Clinton (when asked how she coped with the election loss, she responded by demonstrated alternate nostril breathing), yogi's have been practicing this breathing technique for hundreds of years.

This breathing exercise is also the most effective in giving me 'yoga brain' - what yoga practitioners refer to as the feeling of being both relaxed and alert. This exercise can give you a burst of energy, help you feel calm, and enhance your mental functioning.

How to do it:

- Sit in a comfortable position on a chair or the floor.
- Place your left hand on your knee. With your right hand, extend the thumb and ring finger.

- Place the thumb just over your right nostril, and your ring finger just over the left.

- To begin, close the left nostril with your finger, and inhale through the right. Hold the breath while you release the left nostril and cover the right. Exhale through the left nostril.

- On your next inhale breathe through the left nostril. Hold the breath as you switch fingers, and exhale through the right.

- Continue for 3-5 minutes.

Bee breath

Many people find the bee breath (officially known as brahmari) helps with anxiety. Since chronic pain can cause feelings of anxiety, I find it a helpful practice - particularly before bed or anytime you're feeling stressed out. As the name implies, this exercise requires making a buzzing noise as you breathe out. Thus, it's best to do this practice in your own home rather than in public. I've been known to practice alternate nostril breathing in the office or cafe, but I'll save bee breath for when I'm at home.

How to do it:

- Sit in a comfortable position on the floor or in a chair. Begin breathing through the nose.
- After your next inhale, make an extended MMMMM sound as you exhale, just as the last syllable in the OM chant. When you are all out of breath to exhale, inhale, and repeat.

What does the science say about Pranayama?

While the effects of a specific kind of pranayama have not been studied, there is some research to indicate that breathing through your nose, and diaphragmatic breathing, both reduce stress and activate the parasympathetic nervous system. Two studies have found that pranayama reduced heart rate and blood pressure after practicing for just 15 days![vi]

Yoga Nidra

Yoga nidra, or yogic sleep, is a meditation practice that helps you cultivate a sense of safety and wellbeing. It is best practiced after doing pranayama.

I was several years into my yoga practice before I tried yoga nidra. I was sceptical because I had found so much relief from mindfulness meditation. Why should I learn something new if I already had something that was working well? But now, not only do I love my yoga nidra practice; I can see the way that it helps my students, especially those who have trouble with pain. If you have severe chronic pain, you may find it hard to concentrate in a mindfulness meditation because the pain is too intense. However, yoga nidra takes us out of our bodies and cultivate a space away from the stress and pain.

A yoga nidra session of 30-60 minutes can sometimes have the same benefits to the body that sleep has. So, if you struggle with getting enough high-quality sleep, this is definitely a tool you should add to your basket.

Yoga nidra uses guided visualization and imagery to help

students get into a deep meditation. At the beginning of the session, you'll create your own oasis, a place you can visualize in your mind where you feel completely safe and at ease. Then, drawing on these feelings, we can continue through the guided meditation.

Since yoga nidra is a guided meditation, it's not something you can practice on your own. You'll need a recording to help you, or will need to join a yoga nidra class or session in public.

In contrast to mindfulness meditation where we aim to observe, not interact, with our thoughts, in yoga nidra, we welcome thoughts and feelings during the practice. While we still don't judge these thoughts or feelings, we can actively aim to balance them. For example, if you're feeling stress or anxiety, you can cultivate feelings of calmness.

Where do you find these feelings of calmness? Near the beginning of a yoga nidra practice, you will cultivate your inner resource - the safe haven where you feel safe and secure. Throughout the practice, you'll draw on these feelings when experiencing other sensations.

Yoga nidra has recently become popular for people with

anxiety and PTSD, and many programs have arisen to help veterans. I think that this can also be a very helpful practice for those with chronic pain who need a respite from the sensations in their body.

Action Steps

1) Try out each of the pranayama practices. Write down how you feel both before and after doing the practice.

Step 5: Yoga Postures to Relieve Pain

A quick note before starting this chapter: you should speak with your doctor before starting any new physical activity plan. Your doctor can help you identify any potential areas of support that you'll want to discuss with your yoga therapist, or be aware of when starting a home practice. The first rule of yoga is that we don't want to make anything worse. If you have bad knees, high or low blood pressure, or anything else that may affect your yoga practice, you should talk with your doctor to discuss if there are any postures you should avoid, or adapt, in your yoga practice. If

you work with a qualified yoga therapist, they will be able to

help you adapt the poses based on your doctor's

recommendations.

In this chapter, we'll cover two yoga practices - one for the morning and one for the evening. You're welcome to practice these on the same day, or on alternate days. If you're short on time or energy, you can also select one or two postures to do - even if they are postures you do from bed.

Deciding when, and how often, to practice yoga is up to the individual. Traditionally, yoga is practised in the morning. However, the best practice is the one that we can stick to - so I encourage you to find a practice schedule that works for you.

Your yoga practice does not need to last for an hour or more. Even 10 minutes of yoga a day can help you get the benefits of a yoga practice. Studies have shown that people who practice yoga for 10 minutes a day at least 5 days a week have better results than people who do an hour-long practice only once a week[vii].

Yoga and meditation help rewire the brain. In yoga, we call this samskara, and in the scientific world, it's called neuroplasticity. By creating a new habit, we change our brain. The shorter, more frequent, practices are more helpful for making these brain changes. You don't need to practice every day if that is not possible for you, but aiming to consistently practice 3-5 times a week for 10-30 minutes a day can change your brain in the course of a few months.

We need to move the body in all different directions to keep it healthy. In many forms of exercise, such as walking, we're only moving the body in one direction - front to back. In yoga, we move front to back, side to side, and twist, so that the body can explore its full range of movement. More than just the physical, we'll aim to balance the autonomic nervous system in this practice, combining poses that are both calming, and challenging. The first practice focuses on healthily moving the body and focusing on areas of the body that many people report experiencing pain or tension.

Morning Practice

For our morning practice, we'll aim to relieve the stiffness of sleep and warm up the body for the day.

If you struggle to get up in the morning, it can be helpful to lay out the yoga mat in the bedroom or living room floor before going to bed. You can even begin this practice in bed, and then move on to the mat after the first 2 postures.

1. Start lying down on your back in Savasana (corpse pose). Let your feet fall open to either side and lie with your palms facing up. Begin to focus on your breath, aiming to take long, even, breaths through the nose. Breathing through the nose is ideal for deep yogic breathing, but if you're not able to breathe comfortably through your nose, breathe through the mouth.

If you feel yourself drifting off to sleep, it can be helpful to keep your eyes open.

After 5-7 rounds of deep breathing, begin to move the arms. On the inhale, move your arms straight up parallel to the body, like zombie's arms. On the exhale, lower them back down to your side. After 2-3 rounds, inhale your arms completely overhead, stretching them out behind you, and exhale lower them back down. Repeat 2-3 times.

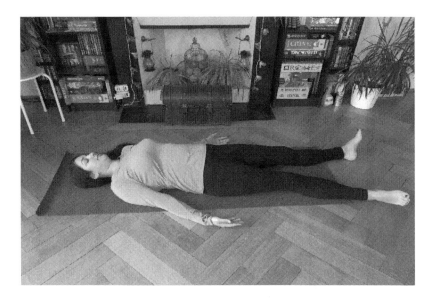

2. Bring your arms back down, and bend your knees to your chest. Wrap your arms around your legs, like you're giving yourself a hug. You can stay still here, or rock from side to side to massage the lower back.

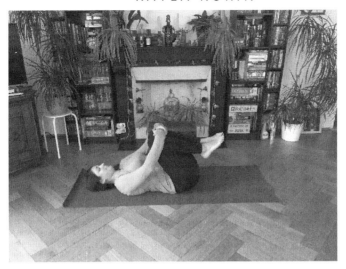

2a. Release the left leg down, and pull the right leg towards the right shoulder. Hold for about 20-30 seconds and then release and switch sides. Then, bring both knees back into your chest and roll onto your side.

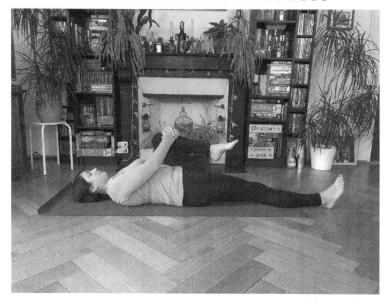

3. From your side, roll all the way onto your hands and knees. Take a couple breaths here to adjust to being upright.

As you inhale, lift your head up, open your chest, curve your spine and lift your hips. As you exhale, drop the hips down, round the spine, and let the head hang loose. Repeat for 5-7 rounds, using your own breath as a guide for how quickly you move. Allow the spine to move fluidly back and forth from cat to cow like a cooked piece of spaghetti.

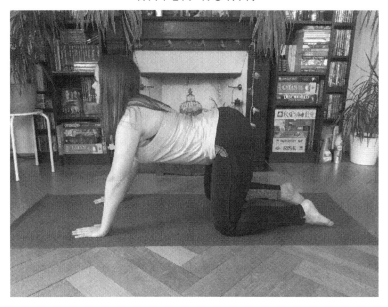

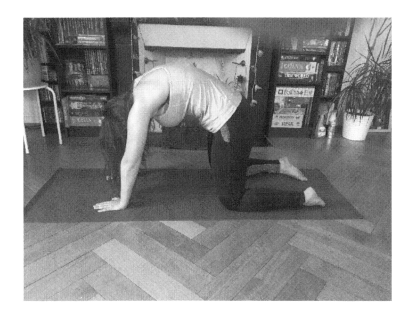

4. Come back to a neutral spine, and then walk your hands

forward until your forehead comes down either on to the mat or close to the mat. Keep your hips over your knees, and enjoy a stretch in the upper back and shoulders. Hold for 5 breaths.

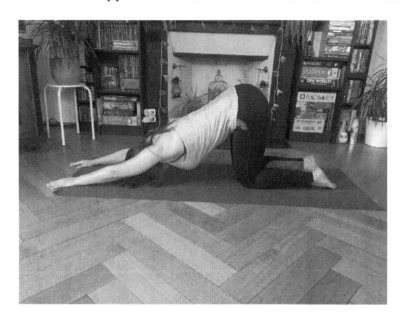

5. Walk the hands back slightly, and curl the toes under. Lift the knees off the mat and stretch the hips towards the ceiling to come into downward facing dog. Hold for 5 breaths. Then, walk the hands back towards the feet and slowly roll up to a standing position. Stand in Tadasana, mountain pose, with the core engaged, for 5 breaths.

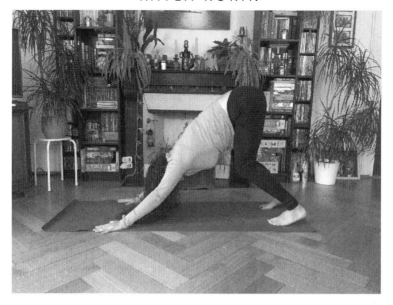

6. Step the left foot back, moving it perpendicular to the mat. The right foot faces forwards. As you inhale, stand up tall and engage the core muscles. Raise your hands straight out to either side. Then, hinge the torso towards the right foot, turning your right hand to your right shin or ankle, and your left arm reaches directly up to the ceiling. Hold for five breaths.

To come out of the pose, look down towards the right foot, and on the inhale, use the strength of the core to come up to centre. Pivot the feet to repeat on the opposite side.

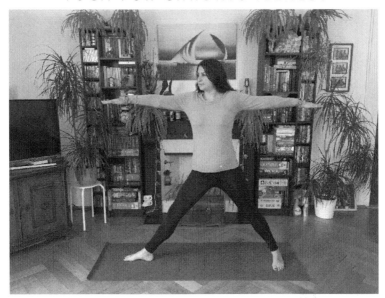

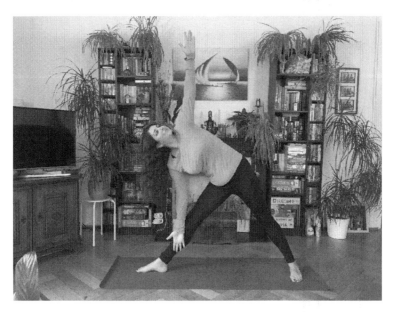

7. Step the feet together at the front of the mat. Take a breath to re-centre before moving to the next pose. Step the

left foot back again, placing it at a 90-degree angle. The right foot faces forwards. Place your hands on your hips to shift the hips forward. If the hips don't move, you can widen your stance by moving your right foot to the right side of the mat. Inhale lengthen the spine, and exhale, bend the front knee, coming into a high lunge. You can either keep your hands on your hips or extend the arms up, coming into a micro backbend. Hold for 5 breaths. To come out of the pose, lower the arms, and step the feet together at the front of the mat. Switch sides.

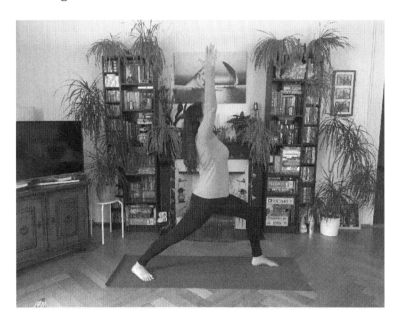

8. Sit down in a comfortable cross-legged position, placing

your hands on your knees. Sitting on a cushion or block if you find it difficult to straighten the spin in this position, or sit on a chair. Inhale to lengthen the spine and sit up tall, as you exhale, move the right hand to the left knee, and place the left hand behind your hips and look over your shoulder. On every inhale lengthening the spine, and on every exhale twisting. Hold for 5-10 breaths, and then switch sides.

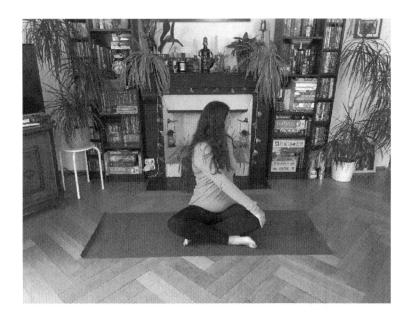

9. Come forward to lie down on your stomach. Slide the forearms in front of you, so that your elbows are beneath your shoulders. If you find this pinches the lower back, slide your

arms forwards so that your elbows are slightly in front of the shoulders. Keep the spine neutral and gaze forwards. Hold for 10-15 breaths.

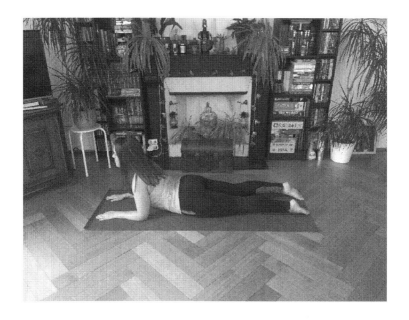

10. Press back on your hands and knees and come all the way back into child's pose. There are two variations of this pose.

10a. Spread your knees as wide as the mat with your feet together. Sit your hips back until your hips reach your heals. If they don't reach, place a cushion or blanket on top of the feet to rest on. Then, walk your hands forward until your forehead reaches the mat. Again, if your forehead does not reach, use a pillow or blanket to support your head and neck.

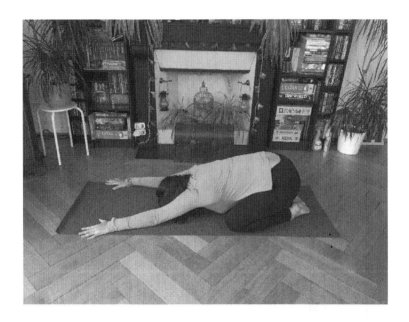

10b. Keep your knees together and sit back on your heels, using a blanket or pillow if your hips are hanging. Then lower your forehead down to the mat, and place your hands, palms facing up by your hips.

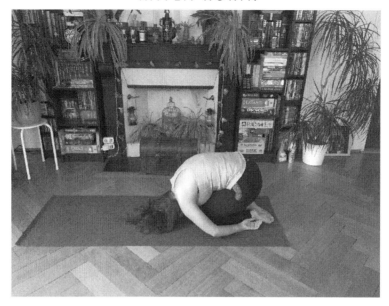

Whichever version of this pose you choose, hold for 10-20 seconds.

End the practice either with a seated meditation or returning to Savasana for several minutes.

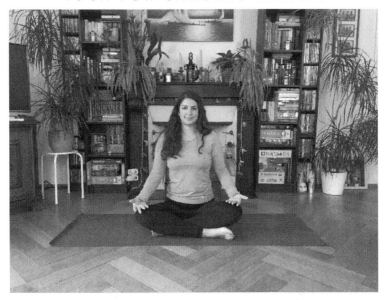

You don't need to do all 10 of these postures every morning, but use these ideas to get into the habit of a short, and regular, morning yoga practice!

Evening Practice

In this evening sequence, we'll focus on releasing tension in the body and relaxing the mind. This is a great yoga practice to do in the evening or before bed. It can also be done in the morning or during the day if you're feeling low on energy.

Because these postures are held for longer periods of time,

many people sometimes find them more challenging than a flowing practice. If you experience any pain or discomfort in any of these postures you should come out of the pose and move on to the next one. If you are able to work with a yoga therapist, they'll be able to help you find an alternative that works for you. However, always remember that you are your own best teacher. You know your body better than anyone else.

If you find that your mind is wandering in these postures, first know that you're not alone. Everyone experiences wandering mind syndrome when meditating or doing yoga. If you do find your mind wandering, acknowledge your thoughts, and then make the choice to bring your focus back to your breathing, letting the thoughts flitter in the back of your mind. It can also be helpful to do some of the breathing exercises or meditations we've covered while holding some of these poses.

For this practice, you'll need a couple of pillows or cushions and a blanket. If you have yoga blocks, those can also be helpful in this practice.

1. Begin in a supported child's pose. Keep your knees

separated with your feet together. Take one of your pillows, and slide it between your knees. Then walk your hands forward, resting your right ear down on the pillow. If the position feels strained, you can use a second pillow.

Hold the pose for 2-5 minutes, and then move your head to the other side for another 2-5 minutes.

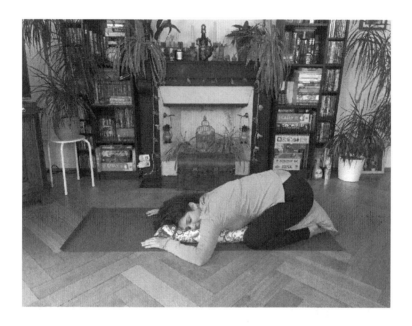

2. Walk your hands up, and come into a normal cross-legged position in front of a chair. Place your hands on the chair, and then rest your head on the chair.

2a. You can have your legs in any position for this posture.

If you'd like to change up the stretch try butterfly (badha konasana) or forward leg bend.

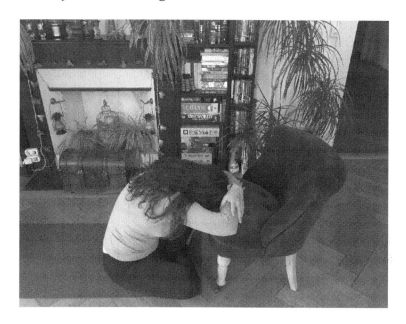

Hold this pose for 3-4 minutes, breathing deeply, and keeping your eyes closed.

3. Slowly come up from this posture, staying in front of the chair. Sitting parallel to the chair (or a wall), place a pillow or cushion behind your hips. Lean back on the cushion and swing your legs up on the wall or chair. Place your left hand on your stomach and your right hand on your heart, feeling the breath moving through your torso.

Hold this posture for 3-5 minutes.

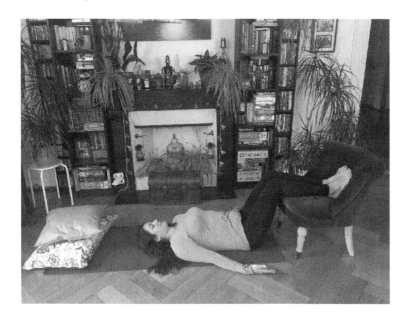

4. Swing your legs off the wall or chair, and move back to your mat for supine butterfly pose Lie on your back, and bring the soles of the feet together. Experiment with sliding your feet backwards and forwards until you find the ideal place for your feet to rest.

4a. To make this pose more comfortable, you can place pillows, cushions, or blankets under your knees to support the legs and hips.

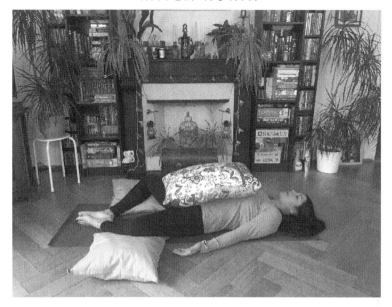

Hold this posture for 3-5 minutes.

5. Stretch your legs out, letting your feet fall to the side, and place your arms by your side with your palms facing up. You might want to place a pillow over your chest under your knees to get very comfortable in this posture.

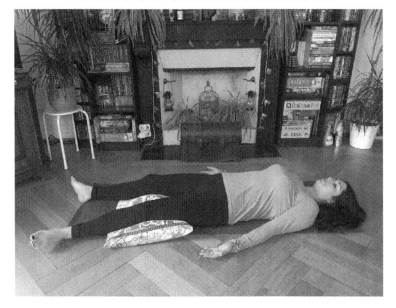

Hold for 5-10 minutes.

You can do these postures before bed or if you wake up during the night and can't fall back asleep. This can help you get back to sleep, or find a place of deep relaxation.

For more 10-15 minute sequences, and to target specific parts of the body such as neck and shoulders, lower back, hips, and hamstrings, check out my 10-day yoga for chronic pain **bundle here, or if you have the print version of this book head to www.arogayoga.com and look under the 'online**

courses' tab.

Yoga During Flare-Ups

A lot of students I've worked with report feeling better after doing yoga for several weeks, but then have a flare-up, and their practice falls away. Once we lose a habit, it's hard to build it up again. Especially if you're in pain.

The good news is, some yogic practices can help you get through a flare. You'll just need to adapt your method to what your body needs. Checking in with your body is a good exercise to do every day, anyways. What you could do yesterday (or 5 years ago) may be very different than what you can do today.

In yoga, we aim to have a beginner's mind. When we first begin to learn something new, we're open to many possibilities. Because we don't have preconceived notions of what the right way to do a new thing is, we can often see many different paths.

As Zen teacher, Suzuki Roshi said, "In the beginner's mind there are many possibilities, but in the expert's there are few."

Because yoga has made it into the mainstream, many people start yoga with preconceptions, making it harder to keep a beginners mind during your practice. This leads many people to feel like they're 'not good at yoga'. We see images of yogi's that are mostly thin, young, flexible, healthy, white women. The reality is there are many different kinds of yoga, yogi's, and yoga practices.

When we remember there is no 'right' way to do yoga or no 'good' way to do yoga, it makes planning for flare-ups easier. Yoga is much more than a physical practice, and checking in with meditation and breathing exercises, can help you find ways to maintain your practice during a flare-up.

The first step in maintaining your practice during a flare-up is to have a flare-up plan. When you have a flare-up, doing necessary things like showering or making food can be a struggle - understandably, yoga often falls by the wayside during these times. However, making a plan now, to commit to a non-physical practice during a flare-up can help you keep your practice up during harder times.

Another helpful tip is to find practices that you can do in

bed. This can be a mindfulness meditation, yoga nidra, pranayama, visualization, or even a restorative yoga practice.

If you listen to a yoga video and visualize doing the actions without actually moving your body, your muscles can still benefit from this. One study found that people who imagined doing a physical practice got up to 70% of the muscular benefits they would get by actually doing the physical practice! [viii]

If you would like to include a physical practice in your flare-up plan, stick to a restorative practice, like the evening sequence in this chapter. You can even pick just one posture from this book to do every day during a flare-up.

I once had a teacher who said, 'the intention to practice yoga, is yoga'. Remember that yogic goal setting is what we can control, not the outcome. You don't need to do a hard physical practice. In fact, if you're having a bad day, you shouldn't aim to do that. You should set a goal to do what is nourishing for your body each day.

Action Steps

1) Set a goal for your yoga practice. How many times a week do you think you can practice? What time of day is best for you?

2) Do it! Set aside the time in your daily calendar to commit to this yoga practice for at least 6 weeks.

3) Make a plan for flare-ups. What yoga, breathing, or meditation practices can you do when you're not up for an active yoga practice?

Step 6: Self Care

Yoga and meditation are great tools for reducing pain and improving your health. There are also other yogic lifestyle changes you can make to improve your health and manage your pain.

Self-care is a broad term and is used to refer to a variety of activities. In this book, I'm looking at self-care from a yogic perspective. What are other yogic things that we can do to improve our health and nourish our bodies?

From an Ayurvedic perspective, chronic pain is an imbalance of the vata dosha. The recommendations in this chapter will help you to balance the vata dosha by creating routines, and finding slow, nourishing activities that counterbalance the flightiness of vata.

Creating a Morning Routine

Creating a morning routine is an integral part of the yogic lifestyle. When I lived in an Ashram in India, the wake-up bell rang promptly at 4 am every day. We then went to a chanting session, to a chai (tea) session, to a meditation session, and then 'free time' where you could practice yoga or use your neti pot*. It wasn't until 8 am, 4 hours after waking up, that we ate breakfast.

I don't expect most people will want to follow a morning routine like this. However, creating a routine that works for your lifestyle can help you wake up with more energy each morning, and clear away the fog of sleep. Ideally, you'll wake up before the sunrise, but if that's not possible, a buffer of at least an hour before you have work or familial responsibilities is an excellent time to wake up.

When you wake up, instead of checking your phone or

thinking about what you need to do, choose a relaxing activity like meditation, or reading a book. From there, you can select some of the suggestions in this chapter to build a morning routine that works for you.

An example of a morning routine might be:

6:30 am: Wake up

6:30-6:45: Breathing meditation

6:45-7:15: Tea, a piece of fruit, reading a book

7:15-7:30: Self-massage

7:30-7:45: Ayurvedic cleansing activity like a neti pot or pranayama exercise

7:45-8:00: Shower

8:00-8:15/30: yoga

8:30: Breakfast

It will take experimentation to find your ideal wake up time and morning routine. Write down what your ideal morning looks like, and adjust as you try out your routine.

*The neti Pot is a small teapot that you can fill with boiling water and a saline solution. When the water cools to room temperature, over the sink, pour the liquid through one nostril

and out the other. Repeat on the other side. This helps keep the nasal passages clear and has been very helpful to me in reducing the amount of congestion I experience. Being able to breathe deeply through your nose can help you feel calmer and relax tense muscles, which can, in turn, reduce pain. The neti pot can help you to clear your nasal passages if they are often blocked, and can even be used when you have a cold to flush the sinuses.

Massage

Working with an experienced massage therapist can help alleviate muscle pain and tension. From an Ayurvedic perspective, you can get an Indian head massage (which involves dripping oils on your forehead), or an Ayurvedic massage, which consists in rubbing warm oils over the body. These massages can be very relaxing and help to balance the doshas.

Getting a Swedish, or deep tissue massage can get deeper into the muscle tissue to relieve pain. Working with a massage therapist who understands your condition is more important than the style of massage you choose.

Most of us can't afford to get a professional massage on a daily or weekly basis. So starting a self-massage routine in the morning can be a helpful way to start the day. I enjoy going for a massage every month or two, but in between, I try to give myself a daily massage of 10-20 minutes each morning, depending on how much time I have.

An Ayurvedic morning massage traditionally focuses on the head and neck, but I like to give myself a full body massage, or, if I'm shorter on time, focus on the areas of the body that carry the most pain and tension. I usually do the massage right before I shower so if you use any oils, you're able to clean the skin after.

The first step to starting your massage is choosing the massage oil. If you have dry skin, use heavy oil such as sesame, almond, or avocado. For sensitive skin or skin that's often red, use a cooling or neutral oil such as olive, coconut, or castor oil. For oily skin, use a light oil such as flaxseed.

Once you have your oil ready, you can heat it over the stove, or use it at room temperature. Begin with your legs, and work your way up your body all the way to your head. There are many different techniques to use for massage. I usually start with a warming rub of the area, then search out areas of tension to apply pressure to. Press into the tight spots for 5-10 seconds, and then massage around the muscle. It's hard to injure yourself or do harm with a self-massage, so really anything that feels good to you can help relieve stress and pain.

If you do see a massage therapist semi-regularly, you can ask for help creating a daily self-massage routine for in-between professional massages.

Food

"You are what you eat" - Proverb

Food can have a significant impact on your health: both positive and negative. I was hesitant to include it in this book because it is such a vast subject, and because it can be emotionally charged for many people.

There are so many different diets (and I specifically called this section food because I hate the word diet) - that figuring out what to eat can be overwhelming. Not to mention the shame-based way we think about diet and weight in modern society.

I do think food can be a massive tool for improving your health. I do not think anyone should feel bad about their weight, severely restrict their eating, or try a new crash or fad diet to try to 'cleanse' or 'lose weight'. One great thing that's come out of my healing journey is that I appreciate my body for what it can do, not for how it looks.

That being said, here are a few of my recommendations on what to eat:

Ayurvedic Food Recommendations

Vata is related to the element of air. When vata is in excess, this can lead to symptoms such as bloating, gassiness, diarrhoea, and constipation. To combat these effects, Ayurveda recommends consuming warm and nourishing foods and staying away from raw foods like smoothies and salads. Stick to warm soups, curries, rice dishes, and cooked vegetables.

Healthy fats and oils are recommended for decreasing vata dosha, and even a sweetener such as honey can be used in a hot ginger tea. Rice and wheat are considered the best grains for vata imbalance, while the best fruits are those that are denser, such as bananas, avocados, mangoes, berries, and figs. Minimize bean consumption, as beans can cause gas. But cheese lovers can rejoice because dairy is recommended for balancing vata!

General Diet Recommendations

Many people living with Fibromyalgia have food intolerances or sensitivities. Finding out what these are and eliminating them (or radically reducing them) in your diet, can help you feel better. For several years, I eliminated gluten and dairy, and restricted eggs. Now that I'm in recovery, I'm able to eat those products occasionally but can feel the negative effects they have on my body when I eat them.

To find out if you have food intolerances, it's best to work with a nutritionist. They can give you a blood test to check for certain allergies and conditions like celiac disease. You can also try an elimination diet with a nutritionist or on your own if you're not able to visit a nutritionist. In an elimination diet, you remove anything from your diet that could be causing you symptoms. The most common things to eliminate are: Dairy, wheat, rye, spelt, gluten, eggs, citrus fruits, caffeine, alcohol, sugar, soy, peanuts, corn, packaged/processed foods, nightshade vegetables, and anything else you suspect may be causing you digestive issues.

You should cut *all* these foods out for 3 weeks. It can take the body that amount of time just to eliminate the food currently in the digestive tract. Some people feel so good after these three weeks, they don't even move to the re-introduction stage!

To finish the elimination diet, try eating one of the eliminated foods on each day, over the next 3-4 weeks. Do not try more than one food in one day. Even if you do not have a negative reaction to a food, do not re-incorporate it into your diet until the end of the re-introduction phase. For breakfast, you should have one serving of the eliminated food, for lunch 2, and dinner 3. Keep a diary of how you feel after eating the food, and the next morning. After trying each food, you can look over your notes and see if any of the foods causing you pain or digestive issues. From there, decide if you'd like to cut any foods from your diet.

If you're unsure of how to improve your diet, the best advice is still: *"Eat food, mostly greens, not too much"* by Michael Pollan. Avoid overly processed or packaged foods, and cut down on processed fats and sugars. Increasing your fruit and vegetable servings to 7 a day can make a big difference.

Baths, Saunas, and Spas

Since the ancient Greeks, humans have been using water treatments to improve health. Before around 400 BC, bathing was mostly for cleansing purposes. However, the doctor Hippocrates (from the Hippocratic oath) believed that many diseases centred around an imbalance of bodily fluids.

The Greeks weren't the only ones with this idea. You may

be familiar with the Japanese Ryokan, Turkish Hammam's, or Finnish Sauna's - all water or steam-based spa treatments originating in different parts of the world.

In 2009, there was a study that found bathing in hot water could be beneficial for relieving Fibromyalgia pain. [ix]

Other benefits of bathing in hot water may include:

- Helping with sleep
- Deep relaxation
- Relaxing muscles
- A supportive place to do physical activity

(moving in the water is easy on the joints)

Also, the relaxing nature of spas can help activate your parasympathetic nervous system, creating a space of healing for you.

More than just the physical benefits, a nice thing about going to the spa is that it's an activity you can do with friends and family that's both fun and good for your health. Going out to bars or restaurants or long walks may not be possible for you right now. But going to enjoy some hot pools and saunas is a fun activity you can do with your loved ones. My best friend and I go to a water spa a couple times a year, and after only 20 minutes of bathing in the different baths and spending quality time with my friend, I feel completely rejuvenated!

Sleep

Sleep is one of the most important tools our body has for healing. Yet, many people with chronic pain conditions struggle to sleep. People with fibromyalgia may have trouble falling asleep at night, staying asleep, and often wake up feeling unrested.

According to sleep specialists, most insomnia is caused by hyperarousal. If you ever lie in bed feeling like your mind is racing and you can't stop thinking, this is hyperarousal. Even if you're exhausted or feel tired all day, your mind can still be in overdrive at bedtime.

Now that we understand the role the Autonomic nervous

system plays in chronic pain, it's no surprise that people living with fibromyalgia also struggle to sleep. If you're in 'fight or flight' mode, this is not conducive to getting a good night's sleep.

Because the reasons for poor sleep are likely linked to some of your other symptoms, everything we've covered in this book will also help you sleep better. All the systems of the body are connected, and anything we can do to help our system relax, will help both reduce pain and improve sleep.

Sleep is essential, but you also shouldn't put too much pressure on yourself to get to sleep. Often, people can feel anxious about not getting enough sleep because they know they will feel worse the next day. This anxiety makes it even harder to sleep. Then you feel even worse the next day, and it creates a vicious cycle.

Just as it's important to create a morning routine, it can also help to create an evening or night time routine. I also like to have a plan for what to do if I can't sleep. This plan often includes doing one of the poses from my evening yoga practice in bed or doing a yoga nidra or body scan meditation.

Depending on how alert I feel, or if I get an onslaught of ideas, I might get up for an hour and do some writing or reading. This is not the best option as you will wake yourself up. But, if now and then you feel like you'd benefit by writing down all the ideas in your head, finishing something you're behind on, or picking up a book, then I say go for it. If this becomes a regular habit, you might want to re-think it. For example, if you struggle to sleep most nights, and most nights you lie in bed with your legs up the wall until you feel tired, that's a great can't-get-to-sleep plan. If once every month or two you decide to get up to finish some work or write down ideas, that is no problem. If you're getting up several nights a week to work, you won't be addressing the root of the problem and will notice a limited improvement in your sleep.

Yoga and meditation can have some of the same benefits on the brain and body as sleep can have. So if you can't sleep, doing a yoga or meditation practice is a great alternative. There's also always tomorrow night - so don't beat yourself up if you're having trouble sleeping.

There is so much to cover on the topic of sleep that I could write a whole other book on it. For now, I'll give you an overview of the top tips from a yogic perspective, and from a western scientific perspective on getting a good night's sleep:

Yogic ideas:

- Grab your massage oil and give yourself a scalp massage before bedtime.

- Eat a warm meal for dinner - avoiding raw or cold foods in the evening or close to bedtime.

- Set an evening routine, and try to go to sleep around the same time every night.

- Try a restorative or yoga nidra practice in the evening or just before bed.

- Go to bed before 10:00 pm and wake up before sunrise.

- Drink chamomile or valerian root tea before bed.

Western ideas:

- Turn off screens (phone, tv, laptop) 2 hours before bedtime. If you must look at your phone, put on a night-time filter to activate 2 hours before bedtime.

- Drink chamomile or valerian root tea before bed.

- Take a warm bath or shower before bed.

- Avoid any stimulating books, films, work, or conversations in the evening and before bed.

- Avoid caffeine up to 6 hours before bedtime.

- Sleep in a dark, cool room.

You don't need to do all these things but can experiment to see what works best for you and create your evening routine. An example of an evening routine could be:

6:00 pm: Warm meal

7:30 pm: Devices off, work for the day finished.

7:30-8:00 pm: Restorative yoga or meditation practice.

8:00-8:30 pm: Take a warm shower or bath.

8:30-9:00 pm: Give yourself a relaxing head and scalp massage with warm oils

9:00-9:30 pm: Prepare and enjoy an herbal tea. Drink the tea slowly and mindfully and perhaps enjoy reading poetry, or a book (avoiding anything stimulating such as an action-packed book or murder mystery).

9:30 pm: Prepare your room for bed, closing all the curtains and lights.

9:45 pm: Go to sleep.

Experiment to find a bedtime routine that works for you. If going to sleep before 10 pm sounds too early for you, try it out for 1-2 months. It can be difficult if you would like to spend time with friends and family in the evening. But, once you have better sleeping habits, it's easier to make exceptions to your routine. For example, I was very strict with my sleep for the first year of my recovery. Then, I started to make exceptions. If I wanted to go out with friends, I might have an afternoon nap, and then go out and enjoy. Instead of feeling guilty, I would re-commit to my healthy sleep routine the next night. You shouldn't have to give up the things that bring you joy - those things also bring a positive boost to your health. But if sleep is something you struggle with, it's worth it to make sleep a priority for a few months to help your body heal. Then, by paying attention to your body, you can adapt your routine to fit in other things that bring you joy.

Exercise

Yoga isn't the only form of exercise that's beneficial to chronic pain. Movement is good for your health, period. But people living with chronic pain and fibromyalgia aren't always able to exercise. Sometimes your symptoms can get worse with exercise. One of the reasons I loved yoga when I first started practising was because it was an exercise I could do that didn't make me feel worse (pretty much every other activity I tried to do when I was first ill made me feel worse).

If you're at a stage where you'd like to add in other forms of exercise, then here are some tips to add it safely to your routine:

Other mindfulness-based exercises like Tai chi or Chi gong

can be great places to explore if you enjoy yoga but want to try something different.

My go-to exercise is always walking. It's good for the entire body and is a low impact exercise meaning it's easy on the joints. You don't need anything to walk (other than a good pair of shoes) and can go as slow as you need to. You can start out walking 5-10 minutes a day, and gradually increase your distance each week.

As you start to feel better, you can add more intense forms of exercise. I like swimming because I used to be a swimmer, and also because swimming is another low impact exercise that's easy on the joints.

I encourage you to experiment with any exercise you like whether it's soccer, dance, running, etc. Start slow, and do each exercise mindfully - listening if your body tells you to stop.

Creativity

While everything mentioned in this chapter will help to soothe the vata dosha, you should also know that vata thrives on creativity. Help soothe the running thoughts in your mind by channelling them into a creative pursuit of journaling, painting, or photography. Taking the time to nourish your passions and artistic inspirations may help bring you into balance. Schedule time to pursue your passion.

Many people with chronic pain find that they're not able to do the things they used to do, or they can no longer pursue their passions. If you can make time to do something you're passionate about, even for just one hour a week, it can make a massive difference to your health. I know it can feel difficult to choose to do something 'selfish' when you have such limited energy. You may feel like you should be doing something 'practical' like cleaning the house or spending time with family members if you have the energy. But it's important to remember that we will help everyone around us, by taking care of ourselves and our health.

Action Steps

1) Create a morning and an evening routine, and commit to sticking to them for 2 months.

2) Pick the self-care habits (along with the yoga and meditation practices) you are most interested in trying and schedule them into your day.

Step 7: Living Mindfully

I am currently the tallest of all my friends. I've also been this height since I was 12. When I look back through my school photos, I tower over all the other students with my poofy hair and 18-inch height difference. I don't remember when I started hunching my shoulders. Perhaps I just had swimmers shoulders - always moving forwards in the pool. Maybe I felt self-conscious about my height and began slouching. Either way, I've had pretty terrible posture since I was a teenager. This lousy posture causes me a lot of pain in my neck and shoulders.

Once I started practising yoga and meditation, my posture began improving. I could feel relief in my neck in shoulders when I sat up straight in a meditation session. The problem was, this didn't often translate to the rest of my day. When I started developing neck and shoulder tension again recently, I realized that despite doing 5-10 hours of yoga per week, it wasn't making up for the other 30-40 hours I was spending hunched in front of a laptop, sitting in bed or on a couch to work.

It wasn't just the physical yoga practice that helps my posture; it's the little decisions I make all day every day. Am I going to sit at the table, or sit on the couch, placing my laptop on the coffee table? If I sit at the table am I going to sit up straight, or lean back in the chair and let my shoulders round? Am I going to commit to sitting straight, or am I going to let stress get the better of me and tell myself I'll work on my posture later, right now I need to get this work done?

When I make too many poor posture decisions during the day, it doesn't matter how often I do yoga, I'll start slouching again, and my neck and shoulder pain will come back. We've already established that a shorter, consistent yoga practice can have more power than one longer practice. It's also the small, micro health decisions we make each day that have a more significant impact on our long-term health than any major overhaul.

Living a yogic and mindful lifestyle isn't only about practising yoga and meditation - it's everything in between.

I can't count the number of times (especially when living in a bigger city), that I went to a yoga class at a studio, felt very relaxed after, and in the 45 minutes it took me to get home felt stressed out again because the commute was busy. It wasn't until I started to bring my intentions from yoga class - to breathe deeply, to show compassion to others, to be present, that my stress didn't shoot back up after my commute home.

Living a mindful life doesn't mean you need to walk around being zen, calm, and compassionate all the time. Just as meditating doesn't mean we need to stop thinking, being mindful doesn't mean we don't experience all the stresses of daily life, it just means we're able to come back to an oasis of calm.

For example, setting a timer on your phone to do nothing for 15 seconds, or do a short breathing meditation for 2-3 minutes, can make a big difference in your stress levels, and how you feel throughout the rest of the day.

Yoga or meditation aren't the only mindful activities we can do. Anything can be mindful from washing the dishes to taking a shower or talking to a friend. We need to choose to be present again and again and again.

We can eat mindfully, savouring each flavour of food. We can travel mindfully, enjoying each moment, experiencing a true beginners mind every new place we go. We can be mindful in our relationships. How often do you talk with friends and family, and you've each got a smartphone on the table? We can put the phones away, the other thoughts of what we're doing later away, and be fully present in our conversations with loved ones.

All these things are small micro-decisions you can make each day, but can have a significant impact on your pain and energy levels.

When we live in the moment, we are ruled less by our automatic reaction to something, and more by the choices we make. We can choose to be compassionate and kind. To ourselves as much as we are to our loved ones. And to those who might 'bother' or 'annoy' us as much as we are to ourselves. We can choose to have gratitude for the things we have, even when it feels like there is so much we don't have to be grateful for. When you're living mindfully, you can choose to be grateful for the taste of food, or the time you got to spend with a friend. You can choose to be fully present during each interaction or life experience. In other words, you can fully show up for your life.

We can also choose to find joy in our lives. To do the things we love. To explore creativity. To watch the ebb and flow of our pain, and know it is not permanent. Despite our pain, we can find the joy in each moment, as it is.

Thank You!

I hope you've enjoyed this book and you now have some concrete ideas on how yoga can help you recover from chronic pain. If you enjoyed this book, I would love it if you could leave a review on amazon.com or goodreads.com. Your honest review will help me get this information out to more people living with chronic pain! If you have any questions about anything in this book, or would like to update me on your progress, I'd love to hear from you at kayla@arogayoga.com!

About the Author

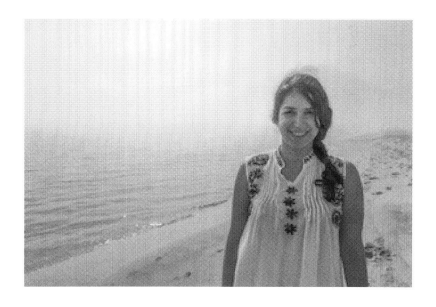

Kayla Kurin is the author of 'Yoga for Chronic Pain: 7 steps to aid recovery from Fibromyalgia'. Kayla is a yoga therapist, writer, and constant traveller who is always ready to embark on her next adventure and share what she's learned with humour, compassion, and kindness. You can learn more about her on her website: arogayoga.com.

KAYLA KURIN

YOGA
— FOR —
CHRONIC FATIGUE

7 STEPS TO AID RECOVERY FROM CHRONIC FATIGUE SYNDROME WITH YOGA

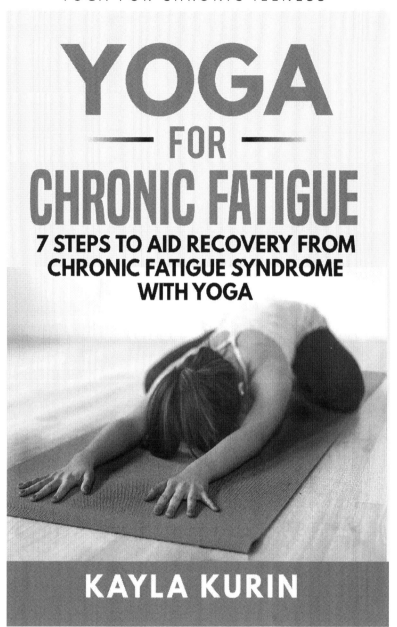

KAYLA KURIN

Yoga for Chronic Fatigue: 7 Steps to Aid Recovery from CFS with Yoga

Kayla Kurin

Yoga for Chronic Fatigue: 7 Steps to Aid Recovery From CFS
with Yoga by Kayla Kurin.

www.arogayoga.com

© 2018 Kayla Kurin

info@arogayoga.com

Cover photography: CC0 public domain
Interior photography: Joshua Schnell

Table of Contents

Dear Reader,

Did you feel tired when you woke up this morning? I know I woke up in pain and fatigue for almost 10 years. The years I was supposed to be "young and healthy" I could barely get myself out of bed in the morning. If you've picked up this book, I'm guessing you know the kind of fatigue I mean. The type of tired where you feel like you ran a marathon the day before, but all you did was switch over a load of laundry. The kind of fatigue where you wake up still tired after a fitful night of sleep. The fatigue that, no matter how long you rest for, doesn't go away.

What's more, there's no known cause or cure for this illness. I know that when I was ill, I was sent from doctor to doctor and had a new bottle of sleeping pills on my nightstand every month, but I never got better. I spent over $1000 on a liquid cleanse when I was a university student and did not have $1000 to spend. The cleanse claimed to be "filled with nutrients" and made promises of: "increases energy!" and "improves sleep!". After wasting a lot of time and money, all I felt was hungry. I still wasn't sleeping, and I still didn't have more energy.

I didn't have, what you would call, a "normal university experience". Sure, there were times when I functioned semi-normally. Times when I went to parties and made new friends to have late night study sessions with. But, there were also the times when my days were filled with emails to professors asking for extensions on the latest paper because of extreme brain fog. There were the hours spent pouring over someone else's notes, trying to decipher what the student hired by disability services had written. There was my boyfriend dropping in for 20 minutes to help me switch over the laundry and pick up a paper to deliver to my professor's mailbox because I couldn't make the 10-minute walk to campus. There were the never-ending doctors' visits. I often wondered what my life would be like after university. Would I be able to have a job? Go travelling? What opportunities would I have had if I wasn't ill and had been able to perform better at school?

While university was one of the lowest points in my journey with Chronic Fatigue Syndrome, it's also where I began my healing journey. From rock bottom, I began to claw my way back to a healthy life.

It was at this time I also got a referral to a new doctor in a holistic health centre. It was here I first started practising yoga and meditation. I also saw a nutritionist, occupational therapist, and counsellor. By making a lot of small changes to my lifestyle and my diet and by getting a fresh perspective on my illness that none of my GP's had given me, I began to get better.

I started to plan for the future, and I was able to get that full-time job (though sometimes had to take short meditation or cat nap breaks!).

At the same time, I was finishing up my psychology degree. A lot of the stuff I was learning in my mindfulness courses, applied to my psychology classes as well. Even if they were using different terminology.

I had spent nearly 10 years waiting for a drug or a cure from my doctors. But my recovery didn't come in that form. It came from years of experimentation and coming to a new understanding not just about my illness but about health and illness in general. It opened my eyes to a completely different world of the body and the mind that has kept me in recovery for the last 8 years.

Creating a mindful and yogic lifestyle opened up a new world for me. I had more energy, I recovered faster from minor illnesses, I took a year-long trip around the world, I ran a triathlon. All things I couldn't have imagined doing a couple years earlier.

I really wish I could tell you that I had a magic spell (energizia!) that could make the fatigue go away. But unfortunately, I don't have that. What I do have is almost 10 years worth of research and experimentation in both western and eastern medicinal practices that I'd like to share with you in the hopes that it will make your journey to recovery a little easier than mine was.

I hope this book will help you better understand your

illness, body, and mind, and give you a variety of tools to manage your fatigue on your journey to recovery. This book is split into seven chapters or steps. The first two chapters are theory heavy and focus on helping you understand chronic fatigue from both a scientific and a yogic perspective. If you're having a brain fog day, you might not take everything in these chapters, but that's okay. The next five steps focus on practical and easy to follow things you can try, and they are the most essential part of the book. As the great yoga teacher, Patthabi Jois, says:

"Do your practice and all is coming."

As a special thank you for picking up this book, you can download a free chronic fatigue workbook to help you track your progress and see which practices work best for you as you move through the book. To get a copy of your journal visit arogayoga.com/chronic-fatigue-journal/

If you're ready to delve into a deeper understanding of how yoga can help you recover from chronic fatigue syndrome — read on!

Sending light and love,

Kayla

Step 1: Understanding Chronic Fatigue

"You may not control all the events that happen to you, but you can decide not to be reduced by them."- Maya Angelou, Letters To My Daughter.

I don't remember everything about the year I started to develop Chronic Fatigue Syndrome. I was so young that it came in a blur. I can only distinguish between the 'before time' because I remember how into sports I was. I swam competitively and was on every school sports team (my favourites were volleyball, basketball, and softball). I had swimming practice almost every day, and for the few years I had been on the team I was steadily improving. Until I wasn't.

I had been excited to go to practices before but now getting in the water after a day of school felt exhausting. My body felt heavy like it couldn't glide through the water anymore. My limbs didn't want to do much more than float. I had never been a morning person but now getting up for school was impossible. I might have stayed up until 4am the night before if I had slept at all (and I often woke up feeling like I hadn't). I would 'clue out' for long periods of the day, not sure what the teacher had said. Or I'd read the same paragraph of text over and over again without taking in any of the information. It was clear that something was wrong, I just didn't know what.

We've all had days where we wake up feeling tired. But if you're living with Chronic Fatigue Syndrome (CFS), you might have forgotten what it's like to wake up without feeling tired. "Normal" fatigue might be relieved by rest, sleep, caffeine, or removing an underlying cause such as a viral illness. Yet, the exhaustion that comes with Chronic Fatigue Syndrome sticks around no matter what treatments sufferers try.

To complicate matters, despite the name, CFS is more than just fatigue. It's persistent fatigue that lasts more than 6 months, is accompanied by decreased mental functioning[x], and often includes symptoms such as joint pain, trouble sleeping (insomnia), sore throat, lowered or heightened immune function, and sometimes depression as a result of the loss of quality of life.

Chronic Fatigue Syndrome has had a controversial history in the medical community. For many years, patients weren't believed about the severity of their symptoms. Even now, many patients are misdiagnosed with depression[xi], or, told it's "all in their head". I was fortunate that over 15 years ago, I got a diagnosis within 6 months. However, after getting that diagnosis, my doctor didn't know what to do with me. I got passed around to different specialists, and yes, often got treated for depression. I was told to drink caffeine if I felt tired or try to push through, and went on a carousel of sleeping pills that never seemed to work for any lasting period of time.

Yet, in the past decade research around CFS has improved, and the scientific community has a better idea of what the illness is. CFS is now classified as a neurological disorder involving the central nervous system (CNS) and peripheral nervous system (PNS). The PNS includes the autonomic nervous system which we'll explore in depth in this book.

While no one knows for sure what causes chronic fatigue syndrome, we do have a better understanding of what this illness looks like in the body. This may help you better understand your fatigue, and also understand how practices like yoga can help you decrease your fatigue. While there are no consistent biomarkers for diagnosing CFS, Anthony L. Komaroff argues in his 2017 study that there are signs that an imbalanced CNS can cause chronic fatigue syndrome. Many studies have found an increase in stress hormones in patients with CFS, as well as reduced levels of antioxidants, and the lack of ability to recover from minor illnesses. [xii]

What we don't know the answer to is the question of: which came first? Do these physiological symptoms cause the illness? Or does the illness produce the physiological symptoms? However, even though we don't know the answer to that question, getting a better understanding of what is going on in the bodies of people living with CFS is helpful to understanding how we can ease our bodies into recovery mode.

Western treatment for CFS is lacking. Since there is no known cause and it's not a life-threatening illness, this illness has not been a priority in the medical community. There are no medications doctors can prescribe to patients with CFS. Depending on your doctor, you may get told something along the lines of, "it's all in your head, see a shrink" or find a doctor who tries to treat specific symptoms like poor sleep without addressing the underlying causes of the illness. If you're lucky, you'll have found a doctor who is willing to take a holistic approach to recovery from CFS.

I do believe that there are many tools we can use from western medicine to aid our healing, and temporary fixes like sleeping pills can be very helpful for people with severe symptoms for the short term. But, in the long run, if we don't fully heal our bodies, we'll have to continue treating the symptoms forever. Some doctors are now beginning to recommend complementary treatments such as yoga, meditation, or massage. But, many patients are left on their own.

While there are some significant gaps in western medicine, specifically when it comes to dealing with a chronic illness like CFS, we shouldn't discount the rigorous research practices applied to western medical practices. We should use these resources when it makes sense to our healthcare team and us. Universal healing strategies like deep breathing, exercise, and diet can be used in conjunction with specific healing strategies like medication or surgery.

I will always refer to my yoga practice as holistic or complementary. It adds to the care I receive from my doctors but does not replace it. I've been able to help many people feel better, sleep better, and have more energy in my yoga practice, but I am not a doctor and don't give medical advice. The most successful cases I've seen are the ones where my student is also working with a physician who understands the power of complementary medicine and meditation.

The Autonomic Nervous System (ANS)

Understanding how the autonomic nervous system works is essential to understanding how CFS manifests in your body and the reasons why tools like yoga and meditation can be more effective than medication. The ANS controls automatic functions like heart rate, muscles, breathing, and digestion. The states of the ANS are referred to as sympathetic (also known as fight or flight) and parasympathetic (also known as rest and digest). When the nervous system is in fight or flight mode, brain functioning is reduced, heart rate increases, muscles tense, breathing shortens, and digestion becomes difficult. Let's take a look at an example of how the autonomic, or fight or flight, system might work:

Imagine that you've gone on a camping holiday, and decide to go on a solitary walk in the woods. While there, you come across a dire wolf, staring at you. You stare back, frozen. Your pupils begin to dilate as you size up the threat, your heart starts beating faster, and your breath shortens as you decide what to do. Should you try to walk away (you don't think this is an option as the wolf starts to snarl at you), should you run for it? Will the wolf be able to run faster than you? Or should you stay and fight? While your brain is trying to make this decision, you might notice you're not thinking about that project due at work next week, when you need to call your mother next, or what you'd like to have for dinner. Your brain is 100% focused on the task at hand. If you do choose to run for it, you'll notice you can run faster and longer than the last time you went for a jog. The adrenaline will give you extra speed and strength. You'll notice your stomach churning and if you tried to eat, would probably have trouble swallowing the food. All your bodily systems are focused on dealing with the threat — and that's a good thing. Imagine trying to think of what time you need to drop the kids at school while facing a life or death situation. Whichever decision you make, your body wants to make sure you have the best chance of survival.

Now, imagine a situation where you're at work, and you get called into your boss's office. Your boss isn't happy with a recent proposal you handed in and wants to discuss it with you. You're new at the firm and haven't finished your probation period yet. As you walk into the office, you might find your body acting similarly to your confrontation with the dire wolf. Your palms might begin to sweat, your heart rate will quicken, your muscles will become tense, and you might get a sense of butterflies in your stomach. Your body only has one reaction to acute stress. Even though you won't need to run away from or fight your boss (at least, I hope so, I don't know what kind of office you work in), your body still responds as if it was faced by a physical threat. And while a call into your boss' office may seem like a big stressor, we're faced with small stressors every day that might set off the fight or flight response. A work email before you get into the office, getting your kids ready for school, getting stuck in traffic or navigating a busy transit system, can set off your fight or flight response multiple times before 9am!

Let's go back to our dire wolf situation. Imagine that, after praying to the seven gods, you choose to run, and make it back to safety. What happens to your body now? You'll probably feel like collapsing. It might take your body several hours to fully relax again. It might even last into the night — you may be afraid to sleep or let your guard down in case the dire wolf finds you again. Most of all, you'll feel exhausted. So, if we're unknowingly activating this system many times before breakfast, is it any wonder we're feeling exhausted all the time?

Finding tools to help balance the nervous systems can help your body heal. When your nervous system is in hyperarousal mode, this is not a conducive state to get a deep rest. Using tools like yoga and meditation to activate the rest and digest system, can help your body work its own healing magic.

When the sympathetic nervous system is activated, you'll notice that:

- Your heart rate increases
- Your muscles tense
- Digestion slows down

- Your breath becomes shallow
- Your palms begin to sweat

If you've ever gotten butterflies in your stomach before doing something you were nervous about, you've experienced the effects of the sympathetic nervous system. If you're living with CFS, you may even feel as though you experience those things on a daily basis.

When the parasympathetic nervous system is activated, you'll notice that:

- Digestions improves
- Your muscles relax
- Your heart rate slows down
- You can breathe deeper

By learning to activate the sympathetic nervous system, we can improve sleep, find more energy, and create a healing state for the body. After all, your body is pretty good at healing itself if only it has the right conditions.

High Sensitivity

Another consideration when thinking about CFS is high sensitivity. The book *The Highly Sensitive Person* by Elaine Aron dives into this topic in depth, and I recommend reading this book if you identify as a sensitive person! I didn't think of myself as a sensitive person before reading this book (I was tough enough to defeat a death eater, indeed), but this book changed my understanding of what sensitivity means.

While it does refer to emotional sensitivity, and it does seem like people with CFS do have stronger emotional reactions[xiii] than the average population, sensitivity refers to a host of things that are out of our control.

Sensitivity may refer to sensitivity to light and sound, sensitivity to people (being introverted), sensitivity to air quality, sensitivity to food, and any other emotional or environmental factors.

If you find that you get drained by city life or being around people quicker than your friends and family, you may be a highly sensitive person (HSP).

This high sensitivity could mean that you're more affected by environmental factors than your peers, which will set off that sympathetic nervous system and leave you feeling drained. Repeating this cycle over many years may mirror many of the symptoms of chronic fatigue syndrome.

While we don't know for sure what causes CFS, we do know some of the related physiological factors that make it harder for us to heal. By using various techniques to soothe the nervous system and build a life that factors in our sensitivity, we can begin on the path to recovery.

Being sick with a chronic illness requires you to become a detective. You need to search for clues to what is making your symptoms worse and be on high alert for the things that make you feel better. By drawing awareness to the things we do know, we can start creating a blueprint to feeling better.

Action Steps

1. Start a journal or spreadsheet to track your progress over the next two months. Make a column to measure your fatigue levels (or any of your other significant symptoms), and start recording times you notice these symptoms intensely. What happened the night before you had a flare-up? What happened an hour before? How long did it last? etc. We'll use this journal to start building awareness of our bodies, and finding what works best for us, as well as what is most harmful.

Step 2: The yogic view of chronic fatigue

"I have been a seeker and I still am, but I stopped asking the books and the stars. I started listening to the teaching of my soul" - Rumi

I'm sitting on a balcony overlooking a sea of palm trees and a wide, winding canal. I'm second in a row of chairs outside the doctor's office. There's a middle-aged American lady on my left telling us she's been feeling exhausted lately and wants to know what's wrong. To my right is a quiet Dutchman who says very little but nods a lot. We're at an

Ashram in the south of India in the province of Kerala, also known as the Venice of India (though I don't think I've seen so much rubbish in the canals in Venice). There's an Ayurvedic practitioner at the ashram that we are waiting to see. The American lady gets called in, and I move up to being "on deck". The Dutchman and I sit in silence now.

I've been reading about Ayurveda at the Ashram (there's an excellent library), and am a couple of years into my regular yoga practice. I want to find out what my Dosha is to see if it provides any insight into my CFS. After another 20 minutes, I'm called into the office. An old Indian lady is sitting there with a notebook. She tells me to sit down but then doesn't say anything as she takes my pulse and feels my skin. In the 40-degree heat, I've somehow managed to acquire a cold, and she asks me if my nose is always stuffy. It is. She scribbles a few things down on a paper to bring to the pharmacy and tells me to avoid showering (or at least avoid getting my hair wet). She also tells me to try not to eat more than one meal a day (an instruction at which I fail).

I'm a Kapha-Vata which means I'm prone to phlegm and fluid build up. I'm not sure what concoctions the pharmacy gives me, but they all taste terrible. However, within a day, my sinuses have cleared. I still have a scratchy throat and feel a bit off, but I'm amazed at the clearing of my sinuses. Usually, when I get a cold, my nose will continue running for weeks after the rest of my symptoms are gone. I didn't gain as much insight as I had hoped into my chronic fatigue syndrome, but I'm starting to think there's something to this Ayurvedic medicine.

What is Ayurveda?

Ayurveda is an ancient medical system that originated in India. Ayurveda differs from western medicine in a variety of ways. Firstly, it's had less rigorous scientific study applied to it. This means you might see recommendations for bloodletting next to diet advice in an Ayurvedic text (though, as far as I know, this is no longer practised in any Ayurvedic hospitals). Another way in which Ayurveda differs from western medicine is that it looks at each patient individually. Rather than trying to find the one thing that works for everybody, an Ayurvedic practitioner will work with you to understand your body type, your diet, your lifestyle, your psychological traits, and any past mental or physical traumas that might be affecting your health. For an illness like CFS, which is a set of symptoms with the absence of another diagnosis, a medical system like Ayurveda is incredibly valuable.

Yoga is just one part of Ayurveda. Ayurvedic medicine focuses on lifestyle, diet, sleep, environment, herbal medicine, and emotional health. Most Ayurvedic patients are given a yoga routine to do based on their Dosha and their illness.

What is a Dosha?

According to Ayurveda, each person is made up of a combination of three dispositions, or Doshas: Kapha, Vata, and Pitta. A practitioner will assess your Dosha and will make specific recommendations based on your body type. This is helpful because you're not getting a "one size fits all" prescription. You're getting the best advice for what has worked for people with similar genetic traits as you. To know which Dosha you are, you should see a qualified Ayurvedic practitioner. However, you can also assess yourself with an online quiz or by learning more about the Doshas and diagnosing yourself. Here is a brief overview of the three Doshas:

Kapha Dosha is an interweaving of the water and earth elements. Content and deliberate, people who have a lot of Kapha in their constitutionsgenerally have a broad, sturdy build, thick hair, and smooth skin.They tend to move slowly and enjoy nurturing those around them. Kaphas will be drawn to slow types of yoga like Yin and restorative yoga.

Pitta Dosha is a combination of fire and water. Fiery and intense, those with a dominance of pitta in their constitution are driven, intelligent, and quick to anger. They often have a medium build with yellowish or reddish skin and red hair and freckles. Because they are competitive and focused, Pittas may be drawn to a vigorous yoga practice like Ashtanga.

Vata Dosha is composed of ether and air. Airy and scattered, Vatas love talking about many ideas and can never seem to get warm. They tend to have a thin build and often have knobby joints. Vatas resist routine and may be drawn to the quick movements of Vinyasa.[xiv]

An Ayurvedic doctor won't make a list of your symptoms and try to fit you in a diagnosis. They'll take stock of your entire self, including your Dosha and your lifestyle routines and habits. They'll then make a personalised diagnosis and treatment plan.

You might be starting to see how a medical system like this is better suited to treating conditions like chronic fatigue syndrome which have no known cause or cure and may present differently in different people.

According to Ayurvedic theory, illness occurs when there is an imbalance between the Doshas. Most people have the disposition to be primarily one or two of the three Doshas. When one or more of the Doshas is out of balance, it can result in disease.

Chronic Fatigue Syndrome is seen as the imbalance of the Vata Dosha, [xv]though it sometimes also involves an imbalance in the Pitta Dosha. In the rest of this book, we'll explore both yogic and western ways in which you can balance the Vata Dosha. If the idea of a Dosha seems to 'woo woo' for you, just think of it as a physiological type.

The Digestive Fire

Agni is sometimes considered to be the fourth Dosha. Agni is the Ayurvedic concept of digestion. In the last few years, many scientists have come to understand the importance of gut health.[xvi]

When Agni is strong, you are thought to be free from disease. If your Agni is weak, your body enters a state of Ama, which means "undigested". If you're not able to digest food you may become weak and lethargic, lack energy, have painful or swollen joints, feel bloated, lack mental clarity, and notice a thick white coat on your tongue in the morning. Do these symptoms sound familiar?

To balance Agni and have a healthy digestive fire, you'll need to adapt your diet, and perhaps start practising Ayurvedic cleansing regimens to help rid your body of Ama and restore Agni to balance.

I talk a bit about nutrition in chapter 6 of this book. However, I recommend visiting a qualified dietician, nutritionist, or Ayurvedic practitioner to develop a diet that's tailored to your body and your needs. If studying Ayurvedic science has taught me anything, is that our bodies can react very differently to the same foods or supplements. If this isn't a possibility for you, I recommend reading the book *Radical Health by* James Lilley for an in-depth outline of different gut healing practices to overcome chronic illness.

Agni doesn't only refer to physical digestion of food but is often also used to talk about digesting thoughts, feelings, information, and emotions. Our body and mind need to work together and find a healthy way to communicate. If we can't do this, perhaps because of ignoring the messages from our body for so many years, or maybe from not paying attention (i.e. Being on your phone while talking to someone or watching a film), it can lead to illness.

Ayurveda teaches us that while finding physical ways to heal is important, neglecting the mental and emotional side of illness is detrimental. Without looking at the whole health picture we are bound to stay stuck in our illness.

The following chapters in this book will aim to help you balance your Dosha and your Agni, and encourage the mind and body to work together in harmony.

Action Steps

1) **Take this quiz** to find out what your Dosha is.

2) Then take **this quiz** to find out which Doshas are out of balance[1].

3) Write your results down, and make a weekly check-in on your Ayurvedic balance.

4) Remember to keep an open mind to the end of this book. See if there is anything helpful for you in understanding your Dosha.

---

[1] Visit yogainternational.com to find both quizzes!

Step 3: Mindfulness as a tool for healing

"Accepting means you allow yourself to feel whatever it is you are feeling at that moment. It is part of the is-ness of the now. You can't argue with what is. Well, you can, but if you do, you suffer" - Eckhart Tolle

When I was first referred to the Mindfulness-Based Stress Reduction (MBSR) course, I was sceptical about how effective meditation would be for me. But I wasn't worried about the difficulty of meditation. Unlike my best friend who struggles to sit still or stop talking even for a few minutes, I was a calm person who enjoyed alone time. How hard could sitting quietly for a few minutes be?

Difficult, it turns out. Somehow, the most natural thing in the world to do -- nothing – is difficult for many people (myself included).

What is Mindfulness?

While the type of mindfulness most of us practice today come from Buddhist and Hindu traditions, meditation and concepts of mindfulness can be found in almost any culture in history. Taking the time to pause and reflect is something humans have been doing as part of their spiritual journeys on earth for as long as recorded history.

In Buddhism, mindfulness is part of the eightfold path to enlightenment. While many associate mindfulness with meditation, The Buddha encouraged his followers to practice mindfulness all the time.

If you're interested, you can read more about mindfulness from your cultural tradition. However, in this book, I'm going to focus on mindfulness from a medical perspective. Jon Kabat Zinn is often credited with bringing mindfulness into the medical setting in the 1970's. Yet, mindfulness practices in the medical system can be traced as far back as the ancient Greeks.

Over the last 50 years, mindfulness has seeped its' way into mainstream medicine. It's been used to aid in cancer treatment, help those with chronic pain and fatigue, ease the stress of palliative care, and help keep people healthier and happier.

At this point you might be thinking, I already spend more time than I want lying or sitting in bed, how is practising mindfulness going to help me feel better?

The difference lies in the way we rest. We often don't rest deeply. I used to think I was relaxing by watching TV or reading a book, but, while doing these activities doesn't put stress on the body or muscular system, it isn't calming for the mind or the nervous system. Now that everyone has a laptop, a phone, a tablet, etc. It's easy to have a source (or two) of stimulation with you at all times. By taking 10 or 15 minutes to rest through meditation or breathing exercises, you can feel better rested and have a better chance of refuelling. If you experience insomnia because your mind is always running, there's a good chance you could benefit from mindfulness.

Primary and Secondary Suffering

To understand why mindfulness can be such a useful tool for those with chronic illness, it's important to understand the difference between primary and secondary suffering.

Primary suffering is our initial reaction to something. For example, if you wake up in the morning and feel stiff and exhausted, that's not something you have control over. This is primary suffering.

Secondary suffering is the extra pain we cause by our thoughts or actions. For example, if you wake up in the morning feeling stiff and tired, and then think "I'm going to feel awful all day." this is secondary suffering. These catastrophic thoughts can make the primary pain or fatigue we're feeling worse.

The effects of secondary suffering can best be understood by thinking about the placebo effect. Every first-year psychology student learns about the placebo effect: patients who receive a sugar pill but are told that it's medication, often have the same recovery rates as those who received the pharmaceutical medication in illnesses like depression[xvii]. Secondary suffering is the opposite of the placebo effect. When you believe that your illness won't get better, or that the pain or fatigue is more intense or constant than it is, this can make your symptoms worse.

Stopping negative thought patterns can be tough because negative thoughts are a normal reaction to extended periods of suffering. It's easy to see why people with CFS feel hopeless. I know that I often felt that way when I was ill. Add to that fact that friends, family, and colleagues often don't understand what you're going through, it can be easy to assume your symptoms will be worse just so you're able to give consistent expectations to those around you. I was ill when I was in university, and I always felt guilty when I had to ask for a last minute extension or rearrange an exam date because sometimes I felt completely fine. Imagining that my symptoms would be consistently bad made it easier to plan for my studies. However, it was not helpful for my recovery. I eventually realised that people are more understanding than I thought, and everyone, no matter how healthy they are, sometimes needs time off or last-minute accommodations for their health.

Since these negative thoughts are natural to us, how can we start to change our thought patterns to support our healing? Mindfulness is a tool that can help rewire the brain. It can help you tune in to the sensations you're experiencing in the present moment, not what your mind is telling you you're experiencing.

The Science Behind Mindfulness

While research in this field is new, the research that has been done on mindfulness therapies are promising for treating or relieving some of the symptoms of chronic fatigue syndrome.

In an eight-week mindfulness study done in 2017, participants showed improvements in anxiety, fatigue, and depression and patients reported an increased quality of life[xviii]. Even after only 2 months of a mindfulness intervention, these improvements were still true in a long-term follow-up.

In 2009, a study was conducted on a body-mind awareness program based off of the MBSR. The study found that the patients showed significant improvements in pain, fatigue, and anxiety. However, perhaps a more important finding is that patients coming out of the program showed higher levels of emotional and physical resiliency, and felt they had more control over their illness and their life than before starting the program. [xixxx]

A different study from 2011 compared Cognitive Behavioural Therapy (CBT), a psychological intervention for people with a variety of illnesses which encourages behavioural changes and managing thought patterns to improve coping mechanisms and Mindfulness Based Cognitive Behavioural Therapy (MBCT) – CBT with mindfulness techniques. The study found that patients showed more significant improvements from MBCT than CBT, particularly those who didn't notice improvements in their symptoms after CBT.[xxi]

Grey Matter

Meditation practitioners and yogi's have always said that they experience boosts in cognitive functioning outside of just a meditation practice. For example, if I meditate in the morning, I feel more focused throughout the day, even though my meditation practice was only 15 minutes. However, yogi's didn't know why this was, and many in the scientific community were sceptical about the powers of meditation. Scientists finally decided to study this phenomenon, and in 2011 a landmark study showed not only that meditation and yoga practitioners were right – the benefits of meditation were present long after the meditation session ended – but there were noticeable differences in the brain structures of yogi's vs non-yogi's.

Remember our friend the central nervous system (CNS)? Let's go back to her for a moment. One of the principal matters that make up the CNS is called grey matter. Grey matter helps to process information in the brain. The amount of grey matter in a given area of the brain affects the functioning of different things such as focus, memory, and stress. The density of your grey matter is determined by your genes, and also environmental factors such as your school environment, alcohol or drug use, and apparently, meditation. In this study from Harvard University[xxii] they found that long-term meditators had more grey matter in the areas of the brain associated with memory, focus, learning, compassion, and self-awareness and less in the area associated with stress. The great news was these results were replicated after participants completed an eight-week MBSR program. You don't need to meditate for years to change your brain, it only takes a few weeks!

In yoga, there is a concept called Samskara which indicates changing the brain or changing behaviour, through repeated action. This is similar to the idea of neuroplasticity in science which says that contrary to what we used to believe about the brain being static after around age 27, we can change our mind by changing our actions or our environment.

One thing I love about meditation is that it only requires sitting or lying down. No matter how severe your fatigue is, you can practice meditation. This is why I've put it as the first practice in this book – it is a great place to start, and a great place to return to on tougher days.

We now know that meditation can help us relax and reduce stress and negative thought patterns. We also know it can change our brain structure to increase cognitive functioning. But, as I said at the beginning of this book, the most important thing is not to read about meditation, but to do it! Here are a few of my favourite meditation and mindfulness techniques to help start your meditation practice:

1. Body Scan

The body scan can be done lying down or seated and can take anywhere from 10-45 minutes depending on how much time you have. I'd recommend setting aside the time for at least one 45-minute practice so you can see what the full scan feels like. Then, make a regular commitment to shorter practices. The body scan helps build awareness of what's going on in your body, without bringing judgement or trying to change anything. The body scan is a powerful mindfulness tool that can help you build focus and awareness. You can practice the body scan with a recording, or on your own.

How to do it:

Lie down in a comfortable position free from distractions.
Begin by taking a few deep, even, breaths.
On your next inhale, imagine that your breath is moving out the bottom of your ribcage, down your legs, and all the way down to your toes. Bring your complete mental attention to the toes, the bottom of the feet, the heels, and the ankles.
Take a few breaths focusing on this part of the body, and then, after a few minutes, release your attention from this area.
As you inhale again, move your attention to your ankles, calves, and shins. Continue the practice by moving your awareness up your body every few breaths.
Notice how you feel in each area of the body, but withhold judging sensations as good or bad. Allow each feeling to reside in your body, as it is.
Once you reach the top of your head, see if you can hold your entire body in awareness for a few minutes (I often like to imagine someone is pouring a warm bucket of water over my head as my awareness expands from the top of my head to the tip of my toes).

To come out of the practice, bring your awareness back to your breathing. After a few rounds of breath, open your eyes.

2. Visualization

Visualization is one of the most potent tools for chronic fatigue syndrome. In this meditation, we'll be using visualisation as a tool to build awareness of our bodies, and allow our minds to relax deeply. This practice takes around 10 minutes.

How to do it:

- Lie or sit down in a comfortable position in a quiet place free from distractions.
- Begin to take slow, deep, even breaths.
- After a few rounds of breathing, start to follow your breath with your mind's eye. As you inhale, visualise the breath moving in through the nostrils, down the back of the throat, through the lungs, and into the diaphragm.
- As you exhale, imagine the breath going back through the rib cage, up the throat, through the nostrils, and back out into the room.
- Continue this exercise for 10-15 rounds of breath. To come out of the meditation, take a few final deep breaths, and open your eyes.

3. Awareness meditation

The awareness meditation can be done anywhere – even

in a park outside or a noisy room! The goal of the awareness meditation is to allow all your senses to activate. The awareness meditation is usually done for 5-15 minutes, though you're welcome to do it for longer!

How to do it:

1. Sit or lie down in a comfortable position. Begin by focusing on your breathing. Notice what the breath feels like moving in and out of the body. For example, can you feel the air cooling the insides of your nostrils as you inhale? Can you feel your chest and belly rise on each inhale, and deflate on each exhale?

2. Practice a few rounds of breath with this awareness until you feel focused on the sensations of your breathing.

3. When you're ready, extend your focus to your body. How does the rest of your body feel? Are you fingers touching anything? What does it feel like to be seated or lying on the ground? Is it a hardwood floor? A carpet? A patch of grass? How does it feel to be grounded on this spot?

4. Next, extend your awareness to what you can hear. Is it noisy around you? Are people talking? Are there animals making noise, or can you hear the sound of the wind?

5. After a few rounds of breath, move your awareness to your nose. What can you smell? Perhaps the smell of grass, or fresh laundry or last night's dinner. Maybe the scents around you are strong or subtle. Take a few breaths to focus on your sense of smell.

6. Next, extend your awareness to what you're tasting. Even if you're not eating right now, do you notice any sensation in your mouth? Is there a taste from the last thing you ate? Or perhaps what you smell is making your mouth water (or feel a bit revulsed).

7. When you're ready, move your attention to what you see. If your eyes are closed, perhaps you see shapes or colours behind your eyelids. If you like, you can slowly open your eyes to take in the sights around you. Just be sure to observe these sights as an impartial viewer, without becoming judgmental or emotionally involved.

8. To come out of the meditation, bring your focus back to your breath for a few minutes, and then open your eyes.

4. Loving-kindness meditation

Loving-kindness, or Metta, meditation is not from the mindfulness tradition, but I've included it in this section because I think it is an excellent addition the mindfulness practices. In mindfulness meditation, we try to observe our thoughts and feelings and not interact with them. However, in the Tantra school of yoga, we're encouraged to feel and engage with our emotions in a mindful way. This loving-kindness meditation takes 10 -15 minutes and is a way to increase your empathy and compassion.

How to do it:

- Begin by sitting or lying in a comfortable position, and taking a few deep, slow breaths, focusing on your breathing.
- After a few rounds of breathing, bring into your mind the image of someone who is easy to love. Maybe this is a friend, relative, partner, or child. It can even be a pet. Notice how you feel when thinking about this person or animal. What sensations do you feel in your body? In your chest, your shoulders, and your stomach?
- Keeping this person in your mind, say to them (in your head): may you be safe. May you be free from pain and suffering, may you feel joy.
- After a few moments, bring in to your mind the image of a person who is challenging to love. Perhaps this is a family member you sometimes fight with or someone you have problems with at work. Notice how it feels to be thinking about this person. How does it feel in your body? Then, say to this person: may you be safe. May you be free from pain and suffering. May you feel joy.
- When you're ready, begin to think of a person who is very difficult to love. This could be a person you have a difficult relationship with or even someone that is a political or public figure. Notice how it feels in your body to think about this person. Then, say to this person: may you be safe. May you be free from pain and suffering. May you feel joy.
- Next, extend your awareness to the people around you. Perhaps there are other people in your house or in your building. Maybe extending that awareness to everyone who lives in your neighbourhood. Then extending that awareness to everyone in your city, in your country, and the whole world. And now say to

these people: may you be safe. May you be free from pain and suffering. May you feel joy.

- Notice how it feels in your body to extend this compassion to these specific people in your life, as well as everyone in the world.
- To exit the meditation, do a quick body scan, and then bringing your focus back to your breath, open your eyes.

Action Steps

1. Set aside a time to do a 45-minute body scan. You can find a recorded meditation or even join a local mindfulness group. Be sure to document how you feel before and after the meditation.

2. Add a time to practice each of the other meditations one time this week. Record how you feel before and after in your journal, and then choose which practices you'd like to make a regular part of your healthcare regimen.

Step 4: Using the Breath as an Energy Source

"I took a deep breath and listened to the old brag of my heart. I am. I am. I am." - Sylvia Plath, The Bell Jar.

"Breathe through your nose! The nose!" my middle school basketball coach shouted at me as we ran in circles around the gym. But I couldn't – my nose was chronically stuffed. I was struggling to keep up (I liked shooting baskets, not this running nonsense), huffing and puffing my way around the gym.

Throughout my life, I've struggled to breathe well. As a child, I was a mouth-breather (though I like to think I was never as nasty as the bullies from Stranger Things). I had never thought much about the benefits of proper breathing other than thinking about how freeing it would be to be able to breathe through my nose. I had tried sprays and medication, but nothing had cleared the congestion. It wasn't until my trip to the Ashram in India that I had seen my nose completely clear! But, when I started developing a regular yoga practice, I began to notice that sometimes, by the end of a class, I could breathe through my nose. If I practised in the morning, my nostrils were often free for several hours. By the time I got to the point of doing my yoga teacher training, I could breathe through my nose the majority of the time. What I didn't realise was a big part of this magic yoga nostril clearing had to do with the way I was breathing in class. For example, practising Ujayi breath (also known as Darth Vader breath) is accessible to mouth breathers and can help clear the sinuses. I also discovered other Pranayama exercises that helped clear my sinuses and boost my energy levels. It's hard to separate those 2 things because being able to breathe deeply made a significant impact on my energy levels.

As a teacher, I love Pranayama, because when a student is too ill to practice physical postures, just like meditation, Pranayama is something that can be done without physical movement.

What is Pranayama?

If you translate Pranayama from Sanskrit, it means "breath control". Practising Pranayama simply means practising breathing exercises. However, these breathing exercises can have a profound impact on your health.

The goal of Pranayama is to reduce blockages, so that more Prana, or "life force" can flow through the body. This might be a literal blockage like my stuffy nose, or it could be mental, physiological, or emotional blockages that are stopping the free flow of energy. One of the earliest texts of yoga written by Patanjali describes the practice of Pranayama like this:

"When we practice Pranayama, the veil is gradually drawn away from the mind, and there is growing clarity. The mind becomes ready for deep meditation" (yoga sutra 2.52)

Pranayama has been practised in India since the 5th century BCE and is still practised today. Pranayama focuses on four parts of the breath: inhaling, exhaling, holding breath, and retention (on exhale).

From a western perspective, the breath is a fascinating part of the nervous system. Breathing is an automatic action – if you try to hold your breath, you'll eventually pass out and start breathing again– but it's also something we can control. For example, you can hold your breath for a time, take deeper or shallower breathes, and choose when to inhale and exhale. This breath control can affect the body.

For example, when you're upset about something as a child, your parents will often tell you to take a few deep breaths. If you're in a stressful situation, your breathing will often become short and fast. When you're feeling relaxed, your breathing will become deep and slow. Even those suffering from illnesses like asthma can help ease some symptoms by learning to control their breath. Breath can give you energy, help you relax, and prepare your body and mind for more profound meditation.

The breath is a connector between the automatic functions of the body and the voluntary functions of the body. It's, for this reason, yogi's regard the breath so highly. Yoga is about creating connection, and the breath is the ultimate connector.

When is Pranayama used?

The yoga postures (or asanas) are only one part of an eight-limbed yoga practice. While in the west, most yoga classes focus on the physical postures, the meditations and breathing exercises are as essential to yoga practice as the poses. In fact, yoga postures first started being used to prepare the body for sitting in meditation for long periods of time. The physical practice was to aid meditation, rather than the other way round.

You can practice Pranayama either in combination with physical asana practice, along with a mindfulness meditation practice, or on its own. To start, I'd recommend practising Pranayama on its own. As you get more comfortable with the different types of practices outlined in this book you'll be able to combine the exercises in a way that works well for you. If you tend to wake up feeling groggy in the mornings and don't think you could manage a physical yoga practice, Pranayama can be a great way to start your day. It can help clear energy blockages without doing a physical practice that may be too high energy for you.

What Does the Science Say?

Research done on this topic tends to lump Pranayama either in with mindfulness meditation or with yoga. However, the limited research is promising. There was a study done on patients of pulmonary heart disease, one group was given Pranayama exercises to do at home, while the other was not. Both were instructed to walk for 6 minutes. After 12 weeks, they compared the two groups and found that those who had done the Pranayama exercises were able to walk faster and further in their six-minute walking period. They also reported having a higher quality of life than the group who didn't practice Pranayama.

Pranayama can increase your fitness and energy levels – without getting out of bed! Here are a few of my favourite Pranayama exercises:

Ujayi breath

Ujayi breath is often practised during a physical asana practice as it can help link the breath to the movements. However, it can also be done on its own. Yoga teachers often refer to Ujayi breath as "Darth Vader breathing" as the sound you make when doing this pranayama practice is like the sound of Darth Vader breathing through his mask.

How to do it:

- Begin by breathing normally in and out of the nose.
- After a few rounds of breathing, on your exhale, start to make a "hhhhhhuuuuuhhh" sound at the back of your throat without opening your mouth or using your voice.
- Inhale normally through the nose, and continue making the sound on your exhales.
- If you're unsure how to make the noise, think about how you might breathe if you wanted to fog up a mirror. You can even try exhaling through the mouth in front of a mirror. What sound did you make in your throat to get it to fog up?

Alternate nostril breathing

To do this practice, you'll need to sit up, but you can stack some pillows against your bed frame or wall to lean on if this is too much. I often like to do this before the body scan meditation as it can help clear your head and balance the nervous system to deepen the meditation.

How to do it:

- To begin, sit in a comfortable position and bring your right hand in front of you.
- Lower the middle and index finger, and place your thumb over your right nostril and your ring finger over your left nostril.
- Begin by pressing your finger over your left nostril and inhaling through the right. Then, release the left nostril and block the right to exhale.
- Inhale through the left nostril and repeat this process, alternating sides.

Lion's Breath

This practice can feel a little bit silly, but it's one of my favourite Pranayama practices. It helps clear the throat, and I often find it helps relieve stress, tension, and anxiety.

How to do it:

- Sit comfortably on your knees, or in a cross-legged position with your hands on your knees and your arms straight.
- Inhale through your nose and prepare to exhale through your mouth.
- As you exhale, tuck your chin slightly, open your mouth as wide as you can, sticking your tongue out,

and opening your eyes as wide as you can so they are bulging.
- Inhale through your nose and return to a neutral position.
- Repeat this for 5-10 rounds.

4-7-8 breathing exercise

This is a perfect practice to do before bed if you have problems with insomnia. It can also be done at any point during the day where you feel like your body is in hyperarousal.

How to do it:
- Start by lying down in bed, and exhale all the air in your lungs. Then, inhale for four counts, hold your breath for seven counts, and exhale for 8 counts.
- Repeat this exercise for 10-15 rounds of breath, or until you start to feel sleepy and relaxed.
- If you feel like you're struggling to breathe, you can reduce it so that it is the 4-6-7 or 4-5-6 exercise. As you continue practising breath work, your lung capacity will expand, and you will be able to hold your breath for a longer time.

Action Steps

1.Add time in your calendar to practice each of the pranayama exercises one time this week. Record how you feel before and after in your journal, and then choose which practices you'd like to make a regular part of your healthcare regimen.

2. Experiment with when to do pranayama. Does it feel best in the morning? In the afternoon? Before your yoga practice? After your yoga practice? Add a few different exercises over the next few weeks to find the routine that works best for you.

Step 5: Yoga Poses to Reduce Fatigue

"The practice of Yoga on a daily Basis brings us face to face with the extraordinary complexity of our own being." –Sri Aurobindo

When I was first diagnosed with CFS, I had to give up a lot of the things I loved. One of those things was sports. I had a doctors note to get out of phys. ed (my favourite subject other than English!), and I had to quit the swim team and volleyball team. Only softball remained as it didn't require as much energy, but even this sometimes caused a setback. I missed being active and playing sports, but there was so little I could do without suffering a regression.

Despite recommendations from well-meaning family and

friends, I avoided doing yoga for many years. I liked sports, not group exercise classes. I didn't see how it would provide me with any value. I only picked up the first yoga DVD I did because, as I was browsing the DVD section of a bookshop, I was drawn in by their stylish yoga clothes. I thought it couldn't be that "woo woo" if they had good fashion sense!

A few months after trying that DVD, I mentioned to my doctor that I had started yoga and found it helpful, but was struggling to do anything more than 20 minutes. She looked at the cover, said "Power Yoga? No no, don't do that, I'll sign you up for our class at the clinic on Tuesdays and Thursdays".

Finding a class that was designed for people with illnesses like chronic fatigue syndrome opened my eyes to the benefits of yoga. First of all, I could do a full 90-minute class without feeling worse the next day. I realised that yoga wasn't an exercise class, which was the focus of most of the studios in my neighbourhood. Yoga was a tool to meditate, to rest, and to build strength and energy in my body in a therapeutic way.

I loved finding a physical activity that I could do without making myself sick. As my yoga practice evolved, I was delighted by the way it positively impacted my health. After developing a regular yoga practice, I had the tools at my disposal to not only get in better shape but to manage my mental and physical energy.

I wasn't the only one who found yoga a successful

intervention for chronic fatigue syndrome. Countless others I talked to had also found yoga helpful for boosting their energy levels and, for some, leading to recovery.

What is Yoga?

Yoga means "to yoke" or tie together. When you combine yoga postures with the other techniques in this book such as mindfulness and Pranayama, you'll be adopting a full yogic lifestyle that's based on ancient and modern techniques to improve health. This can help lessen your fatigue and treat the root of the problems that may have caused your chronic fatigue syndrome.

The asana practice that yogi's practised thousands of years ago likely looked very different from the yoga we practice today. Monks used to practice yoga to relieve tension in their body so that they could sit in meditation for long periods of time. Yoga was a tool to achieve greater heights in meditation, not a goal in itself.

In the last few decades, we've started to understand the health benefits of yoga outside of spiritual transformation (or, for other modern yogi's, outside of getting a "yoga body").

The Science of Yoga

There was a study done in 2014 that showed participants who practised yoga, showed significant increases in energy levels and reduction in pain levels[xxiii]. One of the most exciting findings from the yoga world, has been that, compared to walking, yoga provided more benefits to the ageing and chronically ill. [xxiv]Yoga is more effective than walking in improving cardiac function, and people who practised yoga rather than walking showed more significant improvements in mood and anxiety.

We know that any form of exercise boosts your mood, but yoga seems to be more effective than most types of exercise in increasing well-being.

Since the science of yoga is new, we don't know why, exactly, yoga is more effective than other forms of exercise. However, long-term practitioners of yoga agree that linking the movement with breath, and practising the postures mindfully, are likely culprits for why yoga is so effective.

Another reason why yoga may be so effective is that in yoga we move our body in many different directions and different ways. Traditional exercises like walking, running, swimming, or sports often include repetitive movements that don't explore the body's full range of motion and leave many muscle and tissue groups unused. We need to explore a variety of movements in our exercise practices to bring the greatest benefits.

I've designed the routines in this book based off of poses that have worked for me and my students, as well as what the leading yoga researchers have found most useful for reducing fatigue. I'm including a routine for morning and evening which could also be used as higher energy and lower energy routines respectively.

Please note: Before starting to practice these sequences, it's important to check with your doctor about any limitations or restrictions you may have. Remember, we want to use all the health resources available to us to improve our health, and your doctor will help to make sure you 'do no harm' when practising yoga.

Morning Sequence

This sequence can be done in the morning to help wake your body up for the day. It can also be practised in the early afternoon if you are feeling up to a more active practice. This series isn't recommended to do in the evening or at night as it can disrupt your sleep.

1. Child's pose

Begin on the ground with your knees and feet together. Sit back on your heals, and walk your hands forward so that your forehead rests on the mat. If your forehead doesn't reach the mat, use a pillow, block, or cushion to rest your head on. Then walk your hands back beside your hips with the palms facing up. If this is uncomfortable on your hips, you can also place a pillow or cushion underneath your hips.

Stay in this pose for 3-5 minutes focusing on breathing deeply.

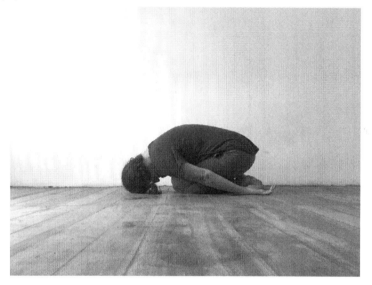

1a. Child's pose flows

On your next inhale, "stand up" on your knees and raise your hands up towards the ceiling. As you exhale, return to child's pose.

Repeat this flow 5-7 times, moving as slowly as you need to and letting your breath guide the movement.

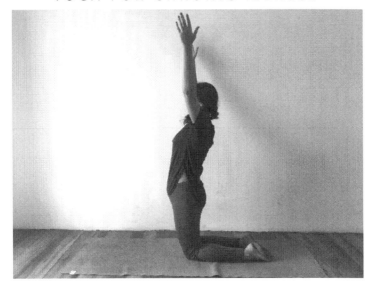

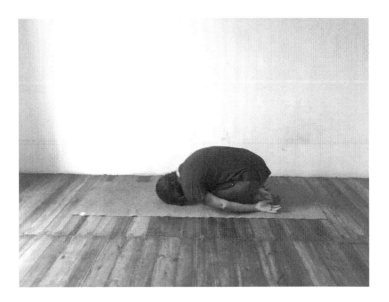

2. Kneeling breathing exercise

After your last flow, come to sit upright on your knees. Here, you can practice any of the breathing exercises in chapter four, or you can try a two-part inhale. Inhale for four counts, hold your breath for four counts, inhale for another four counts, hold for four counts, and then slowly exhale.

Practice this for 2-3 minutes.

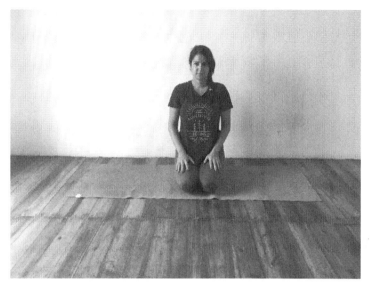

3. Mountain pose

Make your way to a standing position, and stand at the top of your mat. With your feet, hip-width ground the four corners of your feet into the mat. Activate your lower core muscles and roll your shoulder blades back and down the spine. Extend the head and neck as if there was a string that went between the top of your head and the ceiling.

Take 5 deep breaths in this pose, feeling the strength of your body standing tall.

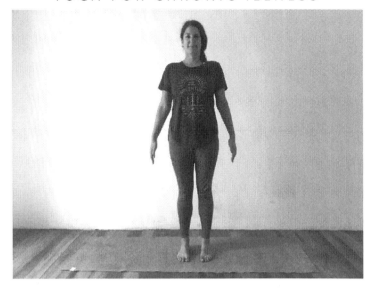

4. Arm lifts

Maintain your strong standing pose. On your next inhale, lift your hands overhead. As you exhale, bring the hands back down to your side, building energy in your body.

Repeat 5-7 times.

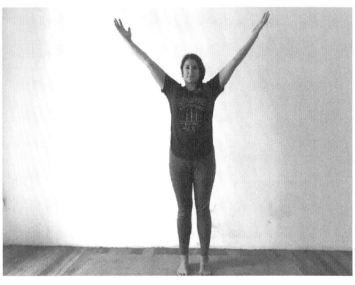

5. Modified forward bend

Inhale to bring your arms up, and then, as you exhale, bend your knees and begin to fold forward until you feel a stretch in your hamstrings. You may want to keep your hands on your hips in a halfway bend or bring your hands down to your shins or behind your ankles.

Hold for 5-7 breaths.

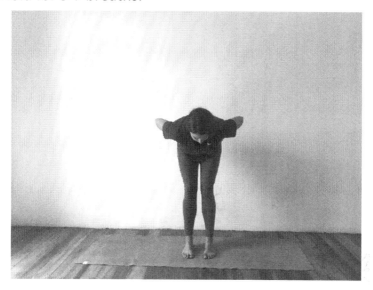

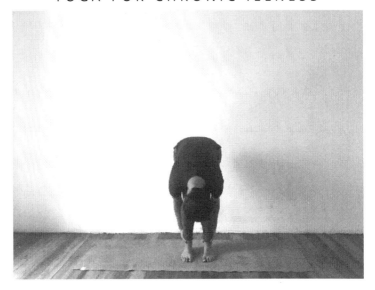

6. Warrior one

Returning to standing, step back with your right foot, placing it on a 45-degree angle. Square your hips to the front of the mat, possibly inching your left food outward to create more space for movement. Next, bend the front left knee, and extend the arms up coming into warrior one position.

Hold this for 5 breaths on each side.

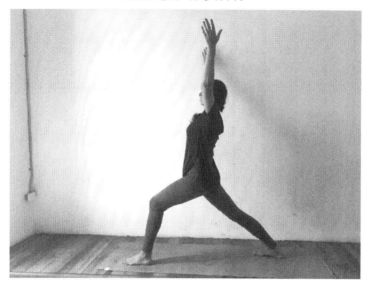

7. Triangle pose

Straighten your left leg, and turn the right foot out, so it's parallel with the back of the mat. Inhale to bring your arms up to shoulder height, and ground through both your feet. On the exhale, "cartwheel" your hands so that your left hand is resting on your left shin or ankle, and your right hand is extending up to the ceiling.

Hold for 5 breaths on each side.

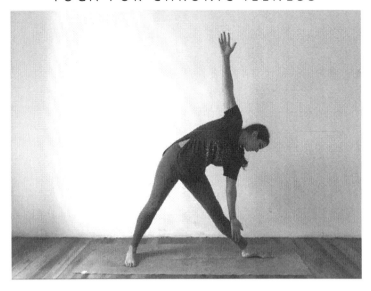

8. Wide legged forward fold

Pivoting your feet to the middle of the mat, keep your feet slightly pigeon-toed and bring your hands to your hips. Inhale to squeeze your shoulder blades together, exhale to bring your hands down to the floor or mat in front of you.

8a. If it's a strain on your back to reach the floor. Use a block or a chair to rest your hands on.

8b. To go deeper into the posture, walk your hands in between your legs, keeping the elbows parallel.

Whichever version of the pose you choose, hold for 5-10 breaths. To come out of the posture, bring your hands back to your hips, and return to standing.

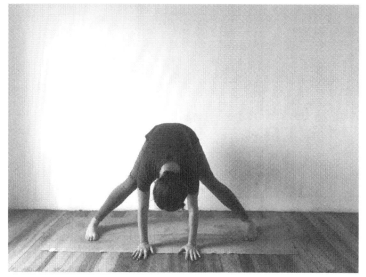

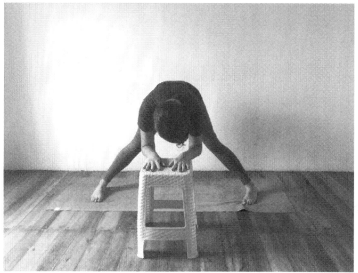

9. Seated twists

Make your way to a cross-legged seated position. If this is uncomfortable, this posture can also be done sitting on your knees or sitting on a chair. Start by bringing your left hand to your right knee, and place your right hand behind you on the ground or on the chair. Inhale to sit up tall and lengthen your spine, exhale to look over your right shoulder and twist.

Hold for 5-7 breaths on each side.

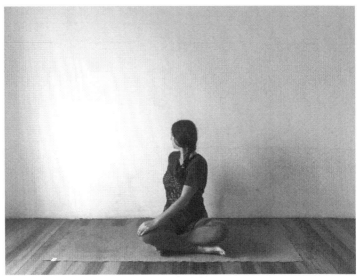

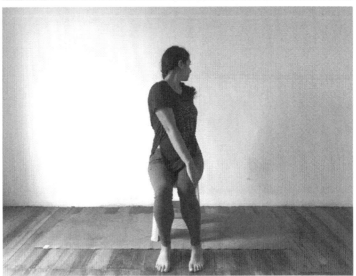

10. Figure four pose

Lie down on your back, placing both feet on the mat.

Bring your right knee into your chest, and then put the right foot just below the left knee. If you feel a stretch in your right hip, stay here.

10a. Loop your hands around your left leg and pull the left leg into your chest to deepen the stretch.

Hold for 7 breaths on each side.

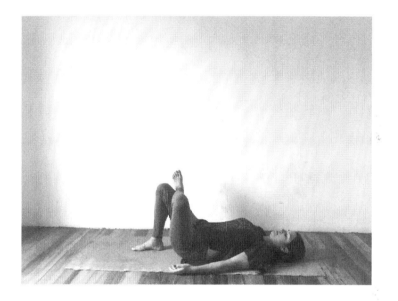

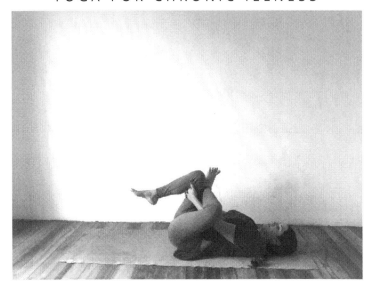

11. Savasana

The final pose of our practice! Extend your legs in front of you, letting the feet fall to either side. Place your arms by your sides with the palms facing up. If you'd like, you can place a pillow under your knees. Focus on your breathing and the sensations in your body.

Stay in this posture for 5-10 minutes, maybe doing a mindfulness meditation practice.

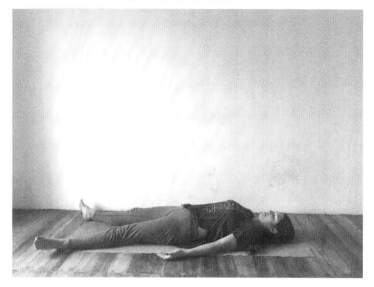

Evening Routine

This sequence is perfect to do in the evening or before bed. Postures should be held for 3-5 minutes to help the body relax and activate the parasympathetic nervous system. If you struggle to get out of bed in the morning, this sequence can also be beneficial to do in the mornings, or any time you're having a low energy day.

If you're lying awake in bed and can't fall asleep, or if you wake up in the night, it can be helpful to do one of these postures until you feel like falling asleep.

1. Passive forward fold

Sit in a cross-legged position and stack a couple pillows on your lap or on a chair. Allow your spine to round as you rest your head on the pillows.

1a. Extend your legs out straight with a bend in the knee and fold forwards.

1b. Sit with the soles of your feet together and let your knees fall out to the side. Again pillows can be stacked on your lap or on a chair.

Hold for 3-5 minutes.

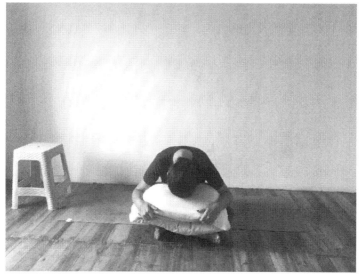

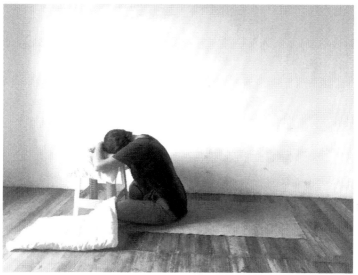

2. Passive child's pose

Sit with your knees as wide as the mat and feet together. Sit back on your heals, and place one or two pillows in between your thighs. Walk your hands forward and turn your right ear down on the pillow. You can also put a pillow under your hips if your hips are tight.

Hold this pose for 3 minutes, switch to the left ear on the pillow, and hold for an additional 3 minutes.

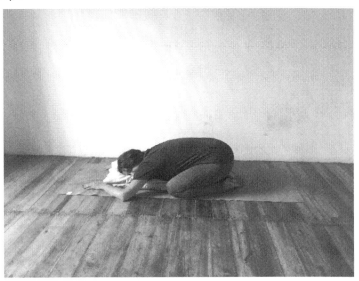

3. Legs up the wall

Lie perpendicular to the wall with a blanket or pillow (if you wish) against the wall. Swing your legs up the wall and shift your hips onto the pillow or cushion. Your legs can be straight or bent, whichever is more comfortable for you.

Hold for 5 minutes.

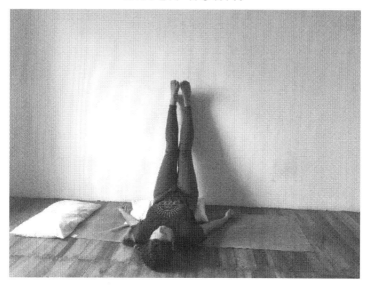

4. Twists

Lie down on your mat with your knees pulled into your chest. Shift your hips slightly to the left and let your knees fall down to the right, placing a pillow between your legs. Extend your arms into a 'T' shape, and look over your left shoulder (or straight up if this strains your neck).

Hold for 3-5 minutes on each side.

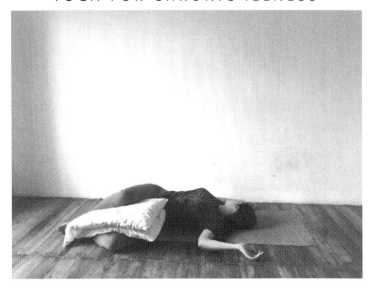

5. Reclining butterfly

Lie down on your mat with the soles of your feet together. Let the knees fall out to either side and place a pillow or blanket under each knee. Rest your hands on your belly or on the floor beside you.

Hold for 5 minutes.

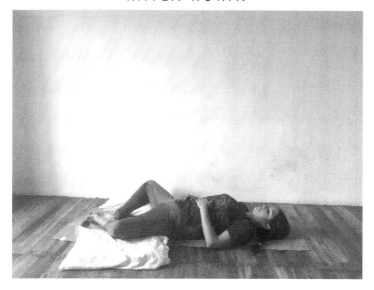

6. Savasana

End this practice by lying on your back in Savasana. There are a few options to use props to make this pose more comfortable. You can experiment to find what helps you feel comfortable and relaxed on the mat. Some options are:

- Place 1-2 pillows under your knees
- Place a pillow under your spine
- Roll a blanket to place along your spine
- Put a pillow over your chest to add some weight
- Pull a blanket over you

You might find one or several of these helpful in finding deep relaxation!

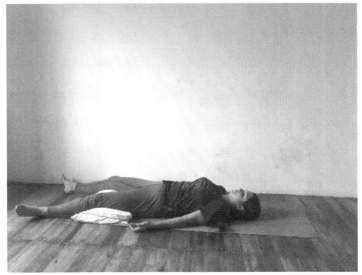

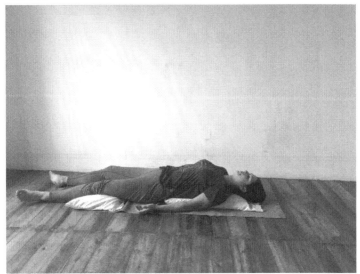

Yoga Nidra

Nidra is a Sanskrit word that means "sleep". Thus, yoga Nidra translates into English as yogic sleep. However, the practice of yoga Nidra is not a practice where you're meant to fall asleep on the mat. It's a practice where you will find a state between wakefulness and sleep which can help you build an awareness of your inner world.

Yoga Nidra derives from the Hindu Tantric school of yoga, though it has roots in several schools of thought in both Hindu and Buddhist traditions. The Tantric school of yoga is a school of thought based on feeling your full range of emotions and finding joy and sensation in every part of life, even the painful bits.

Yoga Nidra is used by yoga and healthcare practitioners for its helpfulness in managing Anxiety, PTSD, and other chronic disorders. Yoga Nidra can help you embrace your thoughts and feelings without feeling trapped or helpless. Yoga Nidra is also beneficial for insomnia. Some yoga practitioners even argue that 45 minutes of a yoga Nidra practice is equal to three hours of sleep!

I love using yoga Nidra as a tool for chronic fatigue syndrome for several reasons. First, many with CFS have trouble sleeping so this can be an excellent practice to do at night when you're tossing and turning in bed. It also doesn't require doing any physical postures so you can practice yoga Nidra even on your lowest energy days. Yoga Nidra brings a deep level of relaxation that can leave you feeling refreshed, which is more useful for building a healing state than reading a book or watching TV.

Like other forms of meditation, yoga Nidra helps release serotonin and decrease cortisol which lowers your stress response. There are also some practitioners who believe that through the progression of the yoga Nidra practice, you move through the first four phases of sleep (leaving out REM sleep). As your brain waves shift from alpha to beta to theta and delta your thoughts gradually begin to slow down, and you're able to notice more about yourself and your current thoughts, feelings, and surroundings.

How to practice yoga Nidra

Due to the amount of visualization required in a yoga Nidra practice, it is difficult to practice on your own. You can use a guided recording or attend a class with a local yoga Nidra teacher in your area.

Yoga Nidra often begins by focusing on your breath and then practising a body scan meditation. After that, the instructor will move into a guided visualisation. This could be visualising a place where you feel safe, a place within your self, or something specific to your instructor and your environment.

As a bonus for purchasing this book, you can try a free yoga Nidra sequence here. If you're reading the print version of this book, send a quick email to kayla@arogayoga.com to get the link to the recording!

Yoga for Flare-ups

Students I've worked with often report feeling better after doing yoga for several weeks, but then have a flare-up, and stop practising. Once we let go of a habit, it can be hard to re-commit. Especially if you're experiencing extreme fatigue and have a limited amount of energy.

The first step in maintaining your practice during a flare-up is to have a flare-up plan. When you have a flare-up, doing basic things like showering or making food can be a struggle. It makes sense that yoga wouldn't be a priority during this time. However, making a plan now, to commit to a non-physical practice during a flare-up can help you maintain your practice and have an easier time during your flare up.

In yoga, we aim to have a beginner's mind. When we first begin to learn something new, we're open to many possibilities. Because we don't have preconceived notions of what the right way to do a new thing is, we can often see many different paths.

As Zen teacher, Suzuki Roshi said, *"In the beginner's mind there are many possibilities, but in the expert's there are few"*.

I encourage you to take a beginners mind to your yoga practice during your flare-up plan. It doesn't matter what you could do yesterday or last month. All that matters is meeting yourself where you are today on the mat.

Many people start yoga with a preconception that you have to be fit, flexible, and thin to practice yoga. If you've been practising yoga for a while and aren't achieving those results, it can feel disheartening or like you're "not good enough at yoga". The reality is there are many different kinds of yoga, yogi's, and yoga practices.

When we remember there is no 'right' way to do yoga or no 'good' way to do yoga, it makes planning for flare-ups easier. Yoga is much more than a physical practice. Committing to meditation, breathing exercises, a bed practice, or yoga Nidra can help you find ways to maintain your practice during a flare-up.

If you would like to include a physical practice in your flare-up plan, stick to a restorative practice, like the evening sequence in this chapter. You can even pick just one posture from this book to do every day during a flare-up.

Another option is to visualize a yoga practice. You can

listen to a video on Youtube or Audible Yoga and imagine your body going into the postures without actually moving. One study found that people who visualized doing a physical practice got up to 70% of the muscular benefits they would get by actually doing the physical exercise!

I once had a teacher who said, "the intention to practice yoga, is yoga". Remember that yogic goal setting is what we can control, not the outcome. You don't need to do a long physical practice. In fact, if you're having a bad day, you shouldn't aim to do that. You should set a goal to do what is nourishing for your body each day.

Action Steps

1. Set a goal for your yoga practice. How many times a week do you think you can practice? What time of day is best for you? Would you like to practice a morning and evening routine every day? Or perhaps alternate days for each routine if time is tight. Remember – the best yoga practice is the one you can do consistently!

2. Do it! Set aside the time in your daily calendar to commit to this yoga practice for at least eight weeks.

3. Make a plan for flare-ups. What yoga, breathing, or meditation practices can you do when you're not up for an active yoga practice?

4. Do you want more variety in your yoga sequence? You can check out this 10-day bundle at www.arogayoga.com/online-courses for a variety of 10-minute sequences for different energy levels.

Step 6: Building Daily Self-Care Rituals

"Change is not something that we should fear. Rather, it is something that we should welcome. For without change, nothing in this world would ever grow or blossom and no one in this world would ever move forward to become the person they're meant to be." – BKS Iyengar

People often ask me what the most important factor in my recovery was. I find this question impossible to answer because I made so many small changes that were important that I couldn't pick just one. I often speak of yoga and meditation, which had a profound impact on my health and my life (I'm writing books on it, after all!), but it's not the whole story.

I spent hours pouring over nutrition blogs and changed my diet. I prioritized creating a healing environment for myself, and my understanding of illness and health changed. When reading recovery stories from others with chronic fatigue syndrome, lifestyle changes are a common theme.

This study from the journal of alternative and complementary medicine includes a case study of a patient with chronic fatigue syndrome. She adopted a yoga-based lifestyle intervention including yoga, meditation, diet, and stress management. After 2 years she reported a significant improvement to her health and quality of life. While lifestyle changes can be hard to measure because it's impossible to account for every individual variation, I don't think recovery is possible without making lifestyle changes.

Your lifestyle needs to support your healing. For example, I often get neck and shoulder pain from sitting in front of a computer all day. Even if I'm doing 1 or 2 hours of yoga day, that can't counteract for the 6 or 7 hours I'm sitting in front of a computer. I need to focus on my posture when sitting, on taking breaks during the day, drinking lots of water, and doing things like self-massage and other forms of exercise to keep the pain at bay.

The same goes for fatigue or any other change you want

to make to your health. Is most of your day contributing to helping you rest and preserve energy? Or is more of your day revolved around spending the energy you don't have?

When talking about lifestyle changes I'm often met with resistance. For some, they maintained certain lifestyle habits for years without getting ill, why should they have to change them now? For others, their friends and family are living a particular lifestyle, and they don't think they're able to make changes and still maintain their relationships. For others, it is merely a resistance to change or a belief that they don't have the energy to make changes.

In this section, I encourage you to make small changes to do your daily and weekly routines. You should spend your time doing things that contribute to healing, rather than things that zap your energy and leave you feeling sick.

You don't need to make every change listed in this chapter. But choose the ones that seem especially relevant to you, and one you feel very resistant to (it's often the things we feel resistant to that we need to do the most), and commit to these changes for eight weeks.

As I've discussed in this book, chronic fatigue is often seen as an imbalance of the Vata Dosha. The lifestyle changes in this chapter are a combination of recommendations from eastern and western traditions, and will all help to balance the Vata dosha by creating routine and unleashing creativity.

Creating a Morning Routine

When I lived in an Ashram in India, the wake-up call came at 4:30am. For those who were brave enough to get up at that time, we'd walk downstairs in the dark for morning prayers. At 5:00am we'd take a chai (tea) break, before going to the beach for a meditation session. After meditation, you were free to practice yoga, go to the library, or contemplate until breakfast was served at 7:30am.

Since leaving the ashram, I don't think I've ever woken up at 4:30 (except for the occasional red eye flight). But, as someone who for years resisted creating a routine, I now feel I have so much more energy and clarity in the day when I stick to my morning routine (which involves waking about around 6:00 or 7:00am, a much more reasonable time).

I said that we often need the things we resist most. For me, this was a morning routine. Especially because I am usually travelling, it can be hard to stick to a routine. But over the last couple of years I have come to value my morning and evening routines. My morning routine helps clear any brain fog left from sleep and eases me into the rest of the day.

My current morning routine looks something like this:
6:30 - wake up

6:45-7:00 - brush teeth, make tea.

7:00-7:15 - journaling/morning pages

7:15-7:35 - self-massage, shower

7:35 - 7:50 - Neti pot* or anything else needed

7:50-8:15 reading and piece of fruit

8:15 - yoga practice (varies in length from 15-75 minutes)

9:00 - breakfast

Your morning routine may look different than mine depending on the activities you prefer doing. Perhaps instead of journaling, you prefer to draw or paint. Maybe instead of reading, you'd prefer having breakfast with your family where you are fully present.

Finding the right morning routine for you will take some experimentation. You can use the above for creating a guideline.

A morning routine and waking up at the same time every day will also help you sleep better at night.

*The Neti Pot is a small tea-pot that you can fill with boiling water and a saline solution. When the water cools to room temperature, over the sink, pour the liquid through one nostril and out the other. Repeat on the other side. This helps keep the nasal passages clear and has been very helpful to me in reducing the amount of congestion I experience.

Sleep

I used to be able to sleep through the fire alarm. At sleepovers, my best friend would get annoyed at me because I would want to stay up late talking. But then when morning came, she would jump on my bed, pull off the blankets, make noise, and still, I would not wake.

When I got sick with CFS, my sleep became awful. I had always been a night owl, but now I was struggling to get to sleep before 3 or 4 in the morning. I couldn't wake up to make it to school at 8:30 so I was always late and had to make special arrangements with my school to continue classes. Even worse than the late nights was the lack of good quality sleep. Even if I slept in till noon, when I woke up, I didn't feel well rested.

Sleep is the most powerful tool we have for healing, so it's frustrating when you're ill, and you can't sleep.

The good news is that there are ways you can improve your sleep without medication. While medication can be helpful for short-term sleep problems (for example, people who can't sleep due to a traumatic event), it's not a feasible long-term solution for those with a chronic illness. It's important to find the root of the sleep problems and address them to have a deep, natural, sleep, rather than becoming dependent on drugs.

I was on sleeping medications for years. The problem was that after 3 or 6 or 12 months, I became resistant to the drug and had to switch. I also wasn't making any of the changes I needed to address the root of my sleep problems. When I started to address these issues, I was able to ease off the medications and get the deep sleep I needed.

The reasons for poor sleep are often related to hyperarousal. However, if you have problems sleeping, you should check with your doctor to make sure the sleep problems are not associated with another condition.

Hyperarousal is a Vata problem; thus all the yoga and meditation exercises, as well as all the changes I'm recommending in this chapter, will help you improve your sleep. In this section I'll make a few sleep specific recommendations, yet, sleep is a huge topic, and I'm only able to scratch the surface in this book.

Western Ideas

When it comes to sleep, there is a lot of overlap between western and eastern ideas. In the west, we talk a lot about sleep hygiene. Here are some sleep hygiene ideas I've found most helpful:

- Stop working, or doing any stressful tasks two hours before bedtime.
- Don't watch scary movies or read thriller/horror books two hours before bedtime.
- Ideally, no screens two hours before bedtime. I know this will be difficult or impossible for many people (myself included). Most smartphones have the option to switch on 'night mode'. Night mode warms the

light on your screen, so it doesn't resemble daylight. Make sure you have this scheduled to switch on 2 hours before your bedtime and last until morning just in case you wake up in the night and want to check the time. You can also download programs for your computer that puts it in night mode in case you need to check something on your computer (or watch Netflix...).

- Avoid caffeine at least six hours before bed.
- Take a warm shower or bath before bed.
- Create a cool, dark sleeping environment, turn off all lights and clocks, and use curtains that block out any light.

As with all the recommendations in this book, you can select the suggestions that make the most sense for your lifestyle.

Yogic Ideas

- Use the massage oil of your choice and give yourself a scalp, shoulder, and neck massage before bed.
- Eat warm, cooked meals during the day, especially for dinner. This means avoiding foods like salads and smoothies in the evening (and perhaps all day if you're really struggling with sleep).
- Do an evening yoga practice. Ideally restorative yoga, yoga Nidra, or a meditation.
- Go to bed within a couple hours of sunset, and wake up before the sunrise.
- Create morning and evening routines and aim to wake up and go to sleep at the same time every day (with slight seasonal variations).

Just like a morning routine can help you shake off brain

fog and prepare for the day, an evening routine can help the body and mind relax as you prepare for a restful sleep. An example of my evening routine is:

7:30 - 8:30pm: Warm, light meal

8:30pm: work for the day done. Most devices turned off. No more exciting television or reading

8:30-9:30pm: restorative yoga practice or meditation

9:30-10:00pm: self-massage

10:00-10:30pm: warm shower

10:30-11:00pm: Prepare and enjoy herbal tea. Drink the tea slowly and mindfully and enjoy reading poetry, positive affirmations, or another book (avoiding anything stimulating such as an action-packed book or murder mystery).

11:00pm: prepare my room for bed, lights out, devices off, pyjamas on, get into bed.

The evening routine you create will be based off your lifestyle, as well as your natural sleep cycles, and the things that bring you joy. For example, my evening routine is about an hour more delayed than an Ayurvedic practitioner would recommend. There are times when I am in bed by 10, but I've always been a night owl. I've found this routine to work for me, and I usually fall asleep before 11:30, as opposed to tossing and turning until 3 or 4 am as I used to when I was sick.

In winter, I'm usually in bed an hour earlier. If I'm teaching a regular yoga morning class (for example, at 8am),

I'll aim to be in bed by 10, so I'm able to be awake by 6:00am and start my morning routine.

The best routine is the one you can stick to, so I encourage you to experiment with what you find works for you. Take a couple weeks to try a few different evening routines, and then commit to the one that makes you feel the most relaxed for 8 weeks.

What to do if you can't sleep

Not being able to fall asleep (or waking up in the middle of the night) when you know you need rest is tough. Unfortunately, willing yourself to go to sleep, or being hard on yourself for not sleeping, has the opposite effect of restful sleep.

If you can't sleep, the first thing to do is accept you are awake right now. Just as wishing your pain or fatigue would go away won't help your symptoms get better, lamenting the fact that you're not sleeping won't help you rest better. There are a few things you can do to increase your chances of falling asleep, or giving your body the rest it needs even if you're not sleeping. Choosing a restorative yoga pose, such as legs up wall, and practising this in bed or the floor next to the bed for 10-15 minutes until you feel relaxed can sometimes be useful in helping you fall asleep. You can also practice a body scan meditation, or listen to a guided yoga Nidra recording. These meditations can help you fall asleep if that's what your body needs. Doing these meditations, even if you don't fall asleep, can provide you with many of the same benefits that sleep can.

If you really can't fall asleep, it can be helpful to get out of bed and go into a different room to do something else for half an hour. For example, reading a book, writing in your journal, etc. Allowing yourself to embrace wakefulness for a little while, as well as leaving the bedroom when you know you can't fall asleep, can help improve your future sleep patterns.

Improving your sleep requires some experimentation and detective work. I hope this section provides a good starting place for improving your sleep and making bedtime a less stressful time!

Food

Food is another topic that I can only brush the surface of in this book. Many people find, as they begin to develop their mindfulness practice, their eating habits naturally improve. As you start to pay more attention to what your body is saying, you'll get a better intuition for the foods that are nourishing for you. Everything that you put in your body: food, cosmetics, creams, etc. enter your bloodstream and can have a profound effect on your health and wellness.

For me, food was an incredible tool for healing. Don't

think of changing your eating habits as "going on a diet". Think of this as a study in nutrition (in fact, I recommend working with a nutritionist or dietician, if possible!) to find the most healing foods for your body.

"Eat food. Not too much. Mostly plants." - Michael Pollan

One of my favourite pieces of eating advice is *"Eat food. Not too much. Mostly plants."* From Michael Pollan's In Defense of Food. Deciding what to eat should be a simple process. We all need to eat food every day to survive! Yet, the modern food industry has made it hard to know what foods are good to eat. Many foods have a health check on them even when the food is something as processed as Kraft Dinner. There are also many foods that mimic healthy foods but, when examining ingredient labels, have a lot of extra ingredients in them that are not so healthy.

The simplest piece of advice I can give is to eat foods without an ingredients label. Fresh fruits and vegetables from the produce section and fresh meat and fish are often the best choices to make. You can also search for dried foods like beans or grains that only have one ingredient on the label (i.e. Rice, chickpeas, etc.). If you're currently eating a diet high in processed or sugary foods, switching to a plant-based diet can have a positive impact on your health.

Food Sensitivities

Many people with CFS have food sensitivities to things like gluten, dairy, eggs, caffeine, etc. If you haven't made any changes to your diet since getting ill, I would recommend starting with an elimination diet. Because we know our whole bodies are working together, and that the gut is a function of the autonomic nervous system, it makes sense that our digestion and our ability to tolerate certain foods can be affected by illness. It's also possible that you've always been sensitive to certain foods, but were able to ignore it or "power through" before. If you'd like to try an elimination diet, ideally you will work with your doctor or a dietician to create a personalised plan. If that's not possible for you, here are the basics of running your own elimination diet:

- Make a list of all the foods you might be sensitive to you. This should include common foods people have sensitivities to such as gluten, dairy, sugar, and caffeine, as well as foods you know you're allergic to, and anything you have an inkling you might be sensitive to. Some other ideas of foods to eliminate are wheat, barley, rye, nuts, citrus fruits, eggs, corn, rice, legumes.
- Cut out all the foods on your list for three weeks. It can often take the body this long to eliminate all the foods from the digestive system. If you're feeling better at the end of these 3 weeks, it's likely you have a food sensitivity.
- For the next 3 weeks, introduce one new food per day. Eat one serving at breakfast, two at lunch, and three at dinner. Write down your reactions to the food that

evening and the next morning. Even if you didn't have a response to the food, do not begin eating it again until you've finished the re-introduction phase.

You should now have a list of foods that made you feel sick after eating them. Cut those foods from your diet.

Ayurvedic diet recommendations

Vata is related to the element of air. When Vata is in excess, this can lead to symptoms such as bloating, gassiness, diarrhoea, and constipation. To combat these effects, consume warm and nourishing foods and staying away from raw foods like smoothies and salads. Stick to warm soups, curries, rice dishes, and cooked vegetables.

Healthy fats and oils are recommended for decreasing Vata Dosha, and even a sweetener such as honey can be used in a hot ginger tea. Other recommended foods for Vata include:

- Rice
- Wheat
- Bananas
- Avocados
- Mangoes
- Berries
- Figs
- Lentils
- Dairy
- Sweet potato
- All vegetables

In both western and eastern cultures, eating a diet that

consists of fruits and vegetables has been shown to reduce the chance of all disease and increase energy levels. If you're going to make just one change to what you eat, I'd recommend increasing your fruit and vegetable servings to at least 7 per day.

Massage

Working with a massage therapist can help many of the symptoms of CFS. It can also help balance the ANS which can contribute to your recovery. Not only can a massage relieve some of the muscular pain that often accompanies chronic fatigue, it can help you stretch muscles that you may be too tired to stretch on your own.

You can get an Indian head massage (which involves dripping oils in a relaxing way on your forehead), or an Ayurvedic massage which consists in rubbing warm oils over the body. This type of massage is helpful for people who are touch sensitive and want a light pressure massage.

Other types of massage such as Swedish or deep tissue massage (my favourite) can get deep into the muscles and joints of the body.

Any kind of massage can help you relax, improve your sleep, and relieve muscle tension. Working with a massage therapist who understands your condition is more important than the style of massage you choose.

Since professional massages can be expensive (unless you have great insurance!), adding a self-massage to your morning or evening routine can be a great way to get the benefits of a massage in-between appointments with a professional therapist. Massaging your problem areas for 10-20 minutes a day with massage oil can release endorphins and ease muscular tension.

The first step to starting your massage is choosing the massage oil. If you have dry skin, use a heavy oil such as sesame, almond, or avocado. For sensitive skin or skin that's often red, use a cooling or neutral oil such as olive, coconut, or castor oil. For oily skin, use a light oil such as flaxseed.

Once you have your oil ready, you can heat it over the stove, or use it at room temperature. Begin with your legs, and work your way up your body all the way to your head. There are many different techniques to use for massage. I usually start with a warming rub of the area, then search out areas of tension to apply pressure to. Hold areas of tension for 5-10 seconds, and then massage around the area. It's hard to injure yourself or do harm with a self-massage, so, anything that feels good to you can help relieve stress and pain.

If you do see a massage therapist semi-regularly, you can ask for help creating a daily self-massage routine for in-between professional massages.

Spas and Water Therapy

One of my favourite activities when travelling is visiting thermal pools, hot springs, and ancient Roman baths around the world! In Japan, I made a point of visiting several Ryokan, and in Bulgaria, I was a regular at the hot springs. I'll take any chance I can to use a sauna or steam room at a gym or health club. From Swedish Sauna's to Turkish Hammam's, different cultures around the world have been using the healing powers of water for thousands of years.

Some benefits of using spa therapies (sauna's, steam rooms, hot pools, etc.) may include:

- Improved sleep
- Deep mental relaxation
- Muscle relaxation
- Fatigue alleviation
- A supportive place to do physical activity (moving in the water is easy on the joints)

Increasing body temperature can help soothe muscles and joints. Also, the relaxing nature of spas can help activate your parasympathetic nervous system.

One thing I love about spas is that it's an activity that's both fun and good for your health. You can visit the spa with a friend or family member and spend time together in a relaxing environment. One of the hardest things about being ill is the hit your social life takes. Having an activity that's both beneficial for your health and lets you spend time with loved ones is a win-win!

Other Exercise

I know that yoga is a powerful tool for managing chronic fatigue syndrome. However, I encourage you to experiment with different forms of exercise and movement.

Walking is always an activity I recommend to my students. Not only is it good for your cardiovascular health, but it helps increase your functionality in day to day life. I also love walking because it's an exercise that's easy to do mindfully.

Start by walking for 5 minutes a few times a week. If this is too much for you, you can start with 2-3 minutes. If you already walk more than that a day you can start with 7 or 8 minutes. As you're walking, avoid listening to podcasts or audiobooks, and focus on the movements and sensations in your body. What does it feel like for your foot to make contact with the ground? How do your muscles feel? Can you feel them shaking and getting stronger? What is your breath like? Can you commit to deep yogic breathing for the duration of your walk? What can you smell on your walk? What sounds can you hear? What do you see? Aim to be fully present on your walk.

KAYLA KURIN

You can walk mindfully either inside or in a park or quiet street. A street with a lot of car or pedestrian traffic can make walking mindfully more challenging.

Other forms of exercise you might want to try are tai chi, chi gong, or any other mindful movement exercises.

Another thing to consider when choosing which exercises to do, is finding movements that bring you joy. Do you love dancing? Swimming? Maybe you can dance for 5 minutes every other day. Perhaps you can go to a public swim and just splash around in the water without swimming laps. There is no better thing for your body and mind than the exercise that brings you joy.

Creativity

The Vata Dosha thrives on creativity. When we get sick with a chronic illness, we have to give up hobbies, or even a career, that brought us joy. Sometimes we may feel like we have to prove we are really sick, and deprive ourselves of joyous things. Other times we may feel like we need to invest all our energy into going to doctors appointments and researching treatments. Or perhaps you feel guilty if you're not using your limited energy to spend time with your family or friends. These are all normal reactions to being diagnosed with a chronic illness. Yet, if we don't make the time to do things that bring us creativity and joy, it can be hard to make a full recovery.

We shouldn't put off doing the things we love until we are well. You can take moments to find joy even when ill. Some ideas for creative activities you can enjoy even when ill are:

- Journalling
- Writing short stories
- Drawing or sketching
- Painting (and the joy of buying new paint!)
- Bringing your camera on a walk and taking photos of nature
- Going to a crafts market and buying yourself a gift
- Knitting or sewing
- Any creative activity you enjoy!

Just as it's important to schedule time for wellness activities in our calendar, it's also important to schedule time for our hobbies! In the action steps, be sure to choose a fun activity to put in your calendar.

I know it can feel difficult to choose to do something "selfish" when you have such limited energy. You may feel like you should be doing something 'practical' like cleaning the house or spending time with family members if you have the energy. But it's important to remember that we will help everyone around us, by taking care of ourselves and our health.

Action Steps

This chapter has covered a lot, and so has a lot of action steps! Feel free to start with just one or two, and add in the others as you find what works for you!

1) Create your ideal morning routine and stick to it as best as you can for the next eight weeks.

2) Create an evening routine, perhaps experimenting with a few different options, and then write down the routine that works best for you and stick to it.

3) Write down everything you'd like to do in the evenings to improve your sleep.

4) Make a can't-fall-asleep-plan.

5) Decide if you'd like to make changes to your diet and then make a food plan.

6) Create a wellness plan. Will you get a massage? Go to the spa? Write it down in your calendar to show your commitment.

7) Schedule a time in your week to do something that brings you joy.

Step 7: Living Mindfully

"The success of Yoga does not lie in the ability to perform postures but in how it positively changes the way we live our life and our relationships." - T.K.V. Desikachar

I'm sitting in a cafe in Ecuador, sipping on hot chocolate, finishing the last chapter of this book. I take a break from typing to bring the ceramic mug of cocoa to my lips. I breathe in the scent of chocolate and then take a slow sip. Made from 70% Ecuadorian cocoa, the taste is a little bit bitter yet rich with aftertastes of vanilla and cinnamon. I look around the cafe and take in the uneven wooden tables and chairs, the hardwood, scratched floor, and the chocolate display table draped with old coffee bean bags. I take a moment to wonder why this "rustic" style is so calming to me. I think it reminds me of being in nature, and thus, I'm experiencing some of the calming effects of being in a natural environment.

I think about how my life has changed since I started practising yoga and mindfulness. I'm not sure I would have enjoyed this moment before I began to bring mindfulness off the mat and into my life. Perhaps I would have chugged down the hot chocolate, wishing it were sweeter. Maybe I would have seen if they had a to-go cup so I could continue rambling around the city. There were fewer moments of stillness. We need these moments of stillness to be present in our lives.

If you've used this book to develop a regular yoga and meditation practice, that's amazing! You're on your way to better health. Yet, the real strength in developing these practices is taking the principles you've learnt into your everyday life. By staying present in each moment, you'll learn to listen to your body and get better at reading the signs about what you need to feel well. You'll feel less pressure always to be doing more, and feel more comfortable doing what you need.

Anything can be mindful. You can put your phone away when you go to dinner with your friends and engage in the conversation. You can wash the dishes mindfully, paying attention to the feelings of warm water, the washing away of dirt. Taking a shower or getting dressed can be done moving with intention.

Once you start bringing mindfulness into your life, you may start to feel like your illness isn't something you have to fight against. Your illness may feel more like an overprotective parent who is only trying to help you do less harm, however misguided their methods may be. You may start to feel like your illness is welcome in your body for the present moment, and that it is something you can work with as you start moving towards optimal health, rather than an infiltrator that needs to be banished.

Making these mindset shifts was so helpful for me in my recovery. It helped me move away from the idea of needing to find a cure to rid my body of disease and move toward the idea of nourishing my illness and body. It was this mindset shift that helped me do the things I needed to for recovery. I started to treat myself like I would a loved one (rather than the over critical not very good friend I was being to my self before), and take the time to heal myself. Even if it meant missing nights out with friends. Even if it meant going home early from family functions so I could go to sleep. Even if it meant creating stricter boundaries with the people around me that I loved. But once I came to love and accept myself precisely for who I was at the moment, those decisions became easy.

I gave myself permission to enjoy moments like these, sitting in a cafe, writing, sipping on hot chocolate.

If you feel good after you practice yoga, living mindfully can help you maintain that for the rest of the day. When I used to live in London, I would often go to a yoga class at a studio and feel great. Then, by the time I got home again I was stressed out because of the busy commute back from the studio. It wasn't until I learned to take these hectic commutes as an opportunity to practice mindfulness, that I started feeling the full effects of my yoga practice.

To conclude this book, I hope you'll set yourself a goal to do one mindful activity a day (outside of yoga or meditation). Eat one meal mindfully with no TV on in the background or book open at your side. Take a shower mindfully, a short walk put laundry in the machine. In time, you can expand to doing more activities mindfully and enjoy the benefits of a fully mindful life.

Action Steps

1) Write down 1-3 things you would like to do mindfully this week.

2) Journal or voice record your reflections from this section of the book, and any part that stood out to you.

3) Write down the things from this book you have found most useful and will now commit to doing for the next few months (or longer).

Final Thoughts

"Yoga does not remove us from the reality or responsibilities of everyday life but rather places our feet firmly and resolutely in the practical ground of experience. We don't transcend our lives; we return to the life we left behind in the hopes of something better." - Donna Farhi

I'm often confronted with misconceptions about yoga. From, "you must be really flexible" to "you seem so calm" and to "I just can't 'turn my mind off' when I try to meditate". Perhaps due to mystic images of Hindu and Buddhist monks hiding away in mountaintop temples spewing out short sentences packed with wisdom, many people think that practising yoga means that you should be calm all the time, and transcend mere mortal things like feelings, emotions, stress, or hardship.

Yoga is not meant to be an escape from life, it's meant to be an opportunity to help you be more grounded in your life. Yoga is not a magical experience that always leaves you feeling serene. In fact, sometimes after I practice yoga, I notice I'm feeling angry or annoyed. These are often from feelings I've been having in my life and not addressing. Yoga practice is not a cure for everything that ails us. Yoga is a way to update your perspective on life by paying attention to each moment, including moments of hardship.

Yoga is not a quick fix or cure. It's something that I still work on every day. It's every small choice I make. To sip my hot chocolate mindfully. To listen to the sounds of the birds and the cars when I go for a walk. To really really try to put my phone away when I'm out with my friends (something that's still a challenge for me at times). Each small decision and small step we take leads to a healthier life, body, and mind. Allow yourself to take your time to explore the different facets of this lifestyle. Why do you need to be in a rush to get well? Instead, can you take this as an opportunity for a time of quiet and stillness with your body? A time to get to know your body, thoughts, feelings, and emotions better so that you can stand by yourself as a supportive friend.

By making these small steps and choices each day, we are slowly treading a path that will lead to better health and a higher quality of life. A path that will open vistas for you to enjoy the small things in life. The time with your friends and family. The time in solitude. Enjoying good food and perhaps a glass of wine.

When we live in the moment, we are ruled less by our reactions, and more by our choices. By choosing to take each moment as it is, we can realize our symptoms aren't constant but ever-changing, and we can live with an open mind and a sense of hope for the future.

Thank You!

I hope you've enjoyed this book and you now have some concrete ideas on how yoga can help you recover from chronic fatigue. If you enjoyed this book, I would love it if you could leave a review on amazon.com or goodreads.com. Your honest review will help me get this information out to more people living with chronic pain! If you have any questions about anything in this book, or would like to update me on your progress, I'd love to hear from you at kayla@arogayoga.com!

To get more information on how yoga can help with chronic illness, sign up for my newsletter at arogayoga.com for the latest blog posts, videos, and courses!

About the Author

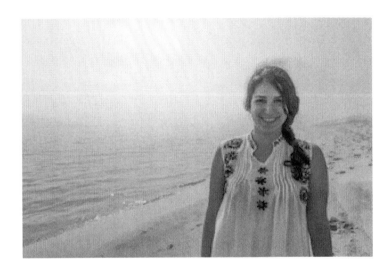

Kayla Kurin is the author of 'Yoga for Chronic Fatigue: 7 steps to aid recovery from CFS'. Kayla is a yoga therapist, writer, and constant traveller who is always ready to embark on her next adventure and share what she's learned with humour, compassion, and kindness. You can learn more about her on her website: arogayoga.com.

YOGA
— FOR —
INSOMNIA
7 STEPS TO BETTER SLEEP WITH YOGA AND MEDITATION

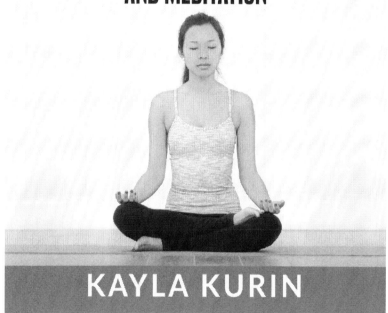

KAYLA KURIN

Yoga for Insomnia

7 Steps to Better Sleep with Yoga and Meditation

By
Kayla Kurin

Yoga for Insomnia: 7 Steps to Better Sleep with Yoga and
Meditation

www.arogayoga.com

© 2019 Kayla Kurin

info@arogayoga.com

Cover photography: CC0 public domain
Interior photography: Shawn Guttman

Contents

Introduction

Dear reader,
You aren't getting enough sleep. You might sleep deeply but only for a few hours a night. Or perhaps you toss and turn in bed all evening, trying to doze off, and never feel refreshed when you wake up. Either way, you find yourself moving through the day in a zombie-like state, not able to be fully present for your friends and family, not able to reach your highest capacity at your job, and not able to enjoy the hobbies that you love.

The okay news is that you're not alone. Around ten percent of the population suffers from chronic insomnia, and thirty percent report struggling to sleep or not getting enough sleep at least some of the time.[xxv]

The not so great news is that sleep impacts every aspect of life. More than diet, exercise, or medication—sleep is the number-one tool that can help slow down the effects of aging, improve and preserve memory, increase athletic performance, help you recover from illness, and have your mind and body functioning at their full potential. The worse news is, those cups of coffee you're drinking? They may cover up some of your sleep deprivation, but they can't match your uncaffeinated brain after a good night's sleep.

The effects of sleep deprivation are so drastic that in Canada alone, the economy loses twenty-one billion dollars and eighty thousand working days due to lack of sleep every year. This may sound bad, but Canada isn't the worst offender. In the United States, it's estimated that the associated healthcare costs that come with sleep deprivation rack up a debt of over four hundred billion dollars annually.[xxvi]

If you've picked up this book, I'm guessing that you wake up feeling tired, have a lack of energy during the day, have trouble focusing, or take longer than your friends to recover from illness. Maybe your insomnia is even a symptom of a chronic health problem, making those health challenges even harder to manage without the restorative balm of sleep.

I've certainly struggled with everything I just mentioned. As a teen, I was diagnosed with chronic fatigue syndrome. Despite feeling exhausted all day, I couldn't sleep at night. I would try to go to bed at a reasonable hour, but I would end up staring at the ceiling instead of sleeping. Once I finally fell asleep, I'd often wake up during the night and struggle to fall back asleep. When I woke up in the morning, I was anything but rested.

During this time, I cycled through so many different sleep medications I can't even remember the names of them anymore. Most of them didn't work. A few did, so I took them for months and months (even when my pharmacist told me I shouldn't be taking this medication for the long term). Eventually, those stopped working as well. I went to sleep test after sleep test, becoming a pro at picking the goop out of my hair from the electrodes. I hopped from specialist to specialist, but nobody could come up with a lasting solution.

I was trying to recover from a chronic illness, but how could I do that when my body couldn't get the rest it needed?

Seven years after the sleep problems began, when I was working with a doctor at an environmental health clinic, he suggested that I sign up for a mindfulness course. I was skeptical at first. If the medications and working with sleep specialists didn't help me get to sleep, how were breathing and stretching going to do the trick? Out of options, I signed up for the course.

In the course, we practiced meditation and yoga and learned about the pillars of mindfulness, breathwork, and mindful movement.

After just a few months of these practices, I started to sleep better. I began to understand the root causes of my poor sleep and how I could fix them naturally without medication, and without being hooked up to any more electrodes.

It's now ten years after I took that mindfulness course, and I've never had to return to medication to help me sleep. I've slept in a noisy, non-air-conditioned apartment in the center of Barcelona in summer, on a train across Canada, in countless creaky guesthouses, and on my quiet, comfortable bed back home.

When you sleep better, not only will you spend less time lying in bed frustrated, you'll heal from illness faster, you'll have less anxiety around sleep, and you'll have more energy for the things you want to do in life.

For me, that means traveling nearly constantly, running triathlons, writing, and taking my niece and nephew to the park.

When I first started these practices, I had no idea what I was doing. If I hadn't had the guidance from my yoga and meditation teachers (and the luck to be living in a place that had yoga and meditation teachers who specialized in insomnia and chronic illness, as well as a doctor who could recommend the program!), I would still be stuck in bed, tossing and turning, waking up feeling worse each morning.

I decided to write this book in a step-by-step format so that what I've learned from studying yoga, meditation, and psychology can help you sleep well without making all the same mistakes I did.

You know how it feels to wake up from a good night's

sleep. Even if it hasn't happened recently—think back to your childhood. The feeling of getting up in the morning with energy and being excited for the day. That's the feeling I hope I can restore to you after you read this book.

As a special thank you for picking up this book, you can download a free insomnia workbook to help you track your progress and see which practices work best for you as you move through the book. To get a copy of your journal visit arogayoga.com/sleep-journal

If you're ready to find out why you're not sleeping well and how yoga can help, read on.

Lots of love,

Kayla

Step 1: Understanding Sleep

My parents love to tell the story of how, when I was four years old, I slept through a fire alarm. My mom was cooking after I had gone to sleep. She burned something and the alarm went off. My brother and sister both woke up and ran downstairs. However, my parents had to come into my room, carry me outside, speak with the firefighter, and then bring me back into my room to sleep, all without waking me. I had been in such a deep sleep that when my brother told me the story the next morning, I thought he was making it up!

Ten years after that incident, when I was a teenager, I couldn't fall asleep in complete silence. Like many teens, I was having trouble getting up in time for school. Yet, unlike my peers who might go to bed a couple of hours later than their parents, I was falling asleep only a couple of hours before first period.

The worst part was, no one could help me. I was referred to a sleep specialist and tried a number of potent medications. I even tried reversing my sleep cycle by staying up all night so I would fall asleep early the following evening, but it never lasted. No one ever looked at the root causes of my poor sleep. Or, if my doctor did, he kept it to himself and continued to try to medicate my symptoms rather than fix the underlying problem.

My doctors had ruled out conditions like sleep apnea to account for my poor sleep, but they had no idea what was causing my insomnia. I had no clue as to what might cause extreme insomnia in the first place. This uncertainty left me feeling powerless, and at the mercy of my doctors. Since I had no idea why I was struggling to sleep, I had to wait for a treatment from my doctor. The treatment was most often a strong sleeping pill that wasn't recommended for long-term use. I didn't make any other changes in my life because I didn't know what types of changes I needed to make.

In university, I studied psychology. My courses helped me understand what happens in the brain leading up to and during sleep. This information helped me know what might cause sleep disturbances. It also began my journey into reading obsessively about sleep and experimenting with my sleep habits.

What happens to the brain during sleep?

At night, you get in bed, close your eyes, and voilà, the next morning, you wake up well rested and ready to take on the day (theoretically). But what is happening to our brains during this shut-eye, and why is it essential for nearly every aspect of our health and daily functioning?

Sleeping and dreaming were some of the things I was most excited to learn about when I was studying psychology at university. So I was a little disappointed to discover that scientists don't exactly know why we need to sleep or why we dream.

However, lack of sleep has been linked to poor daily functioning as well as many illnesses, such as diabetes, cardiovascular disease, depression, and obesity (which isn't a disease but depending on your disposition could put you at higher risk for cardiovascular disease and other illnesses).[xxvii] Sleep deprivation affects memory,[xxviii] reasoning, mood control[xxix]—and it can also lead to death. In the United States, it's estimated that eighty-three thousand vehicle crashes per year are a result of drowsy driving. In a study done on rats, all rats were given a physical task to do, and one group was deprived of sleep while the other group was not. In the sleep-deprived group, many of the rats got sick, were unable to maintain body weight or body heat, and eventually died.[xxx] Lastly, chronically sleep-deprived people (sleeping less than six hours per night) are likely to die earlier than their longer-sleeping counterparts.[xxxi]

Scientists know we need to sleep, at minimum, seven to eight hours a night, but we're still not sure why. However, we do know what happens to the brain during sleep. Scientists have identified five different stages of sleep, creatively named stage one, stage two, stage three, stage four, and rapid eye movement (REM) sleep. REM sleep is when most dreaming takes place. During REM sleep, your heart rate becomes elevated and your muscles become tense, almost like you're awake. We begin in stage one and move down to REM sleep, repeating the cycle every ninety minutes or so until waking up in the morning. Phases one and two are light sleep. When people are in these stages, it's easy to wake them up. People in stage one or two sleep might doze off in a chair and wake easily with a loud noise on the TV. If you're in these stages when your alarm goes off, it will be easy for you to wake up. Phases three and four are the deep, restorative sleep we need to be able to function well throughout the day, heal from illness, and boost immune function. When someone is in these deep stages of sleep, it will be hard to wake them, and they may seem confused or disoriented when they first wake up.[xxxii]

At the beginning of the night, the third and fourth stages (non-REM deep sleep) are most prominent, yet as you get closer to waking, REM sleep takes over more of the deep sleep cycle. If you're interested in how this looks in your brain, I recommend downloading the Sleep Cycle app. You can turn the app on and place it in your bed at night, and it will give you a rough estimate of your sleep stages throughout the night. The app can also set an alarm so that you wake up only in stage one or two sleep, which can help make waking up easier.

Sleep helps us process information, stabilize emotions, and increase focus and energy. When you don't get proper sleep, you may get hungrier and crave sugary foods for an extra energy kick, you may get snappy with loved ones and lose your temper more quickly, and you may be more susceptible to different illnesses. Being able to sleep well is essential to our health and happiness as human beings. So if sleep is so crucial, why is it difficult for so many people?

What are the causes of poor sleep?

There is a wide range of causes of poor sleep, and it's essential to work as a "sleep detective" to try to understand what could be causing this. Seeking what causes your sleep disturbances can help you work with your doctor and take a holistic approach to better sleep and better health. Some causes for poor sleep include sleep apnea, depression, chronic pain, arthritis, restless leg syndrome, allergies, acid reflux, and more. If you've ruled out these other causes, you probably have insomnia, which is defined as:

1. Difficulty initiating sleep. (In children, this may manifest as difficulty initiating sleep without caregiver intervention.)

2. Difficulty maintaining sleep, characterized by frequent
awakenings or problems returning to sleep after
awakenings. (In children, this may manifest as difficulty
returning to sleep without caregiver intervention.)
3. Early-morning awakening with inability to return to
sleep.[xxxiii]

There are also lifestyle causes for poor sleep, such as shift
work and erratic work schedules. Unfortunately, many of our
healthcare workers, such as doctors and nurses, are subject to these
schedules. Shift work can cause a circadian rhythm disorder (also
common in teens), which is when sleepers aren't able to follow a
twenty-four-hour sleep schedule. Shift workers with this insomnia
disorder can sleep enough hours but still wake up feeling
unrefreshed, or they may not be able to get in enough hours of
sleep between shifts. Ironically, the people who are taking care of
our health often aren't allowed to do the thing that can prevent
many chronic health conditions: sleep.

Stress is one of the most significant causes of poor sleep.
The stressors can be temporary, like the loss of a loved one or
losing a job. They can even be positive, like getting married or
getting a promotion. Stressful life events may cause poor sleep for
a few weeks or months, but as the stress passes, your sleep should
return to normal. Yoga and meditation can be helpful tools to
manage stress. If the stress is extreme, medication used
temporarily can help those going through very tough times find
rest. When your stress is chronic, perhaps due to a stressful job,
general anxiety, or supporting a loved one with a chronic
condition, it can cause long-term hyperarousal and sleep issues.
You may dream of getting into bed all day but then be unable to
sleep at night. This is because stress causes arousal of the fight or
flight nervous system. Insomniacs also have higher levels of
cortisol and adrenocorticotropic hormone (ACTH), which are both
stress hormones, in their bloodstreams than those in a control

group.[xxxiv]

The autonomic nervous system and physiological arousal

Many of us use an alarm clock to wake up in the morning. Ideally, we'd all wake up naturally, but the alarm helps make sure that we can get to work, school, and other obligations on time. It's never fun to wake up to the beeping of an alarm clock. Doing so once a day probably won't have a lasting impact on your health and is often necessary to accomplish your goals. Now, imagine that you had to carry your alarm around with you all day, and at random intervals throughout the day, your alarm would go off. You'd probably feel on edge and nervous waiting for it to go off. Each time it went off, you'd probably feel your muscles tense and your heart rate speed up as you searched for it in your bag to turn it off. Instead of helping you accomplish what you wanted to during the day, it would act as a hindrance to getting things done. None of us would want to walk around with an alarm clock that randomly went off throughout the day. Yet this is how many of us live with our internal alarm systems.

Having an alarm that's continually going off would leave your body in a state of hyperarousal. As you can imagine from the example above, it would be hard to fall asleep at night, as part of you would be waiting for the alarm to go off.

To better understand hyperarousal, we need to look at the autonomic nervous system (ANS). The ANS contains your sympathetic nervous system (SNS, also known as fight or flight) and your parasympathetic system (PNS, also known as rest and digest). Both parts of the autonomic nervous system are essential for our survival. For example, if you're walking alone to your car at night and hear someone walking behind you, it's your survival instinct kicking in when you walk quickly, check over your shoulder, and stay on high alert until you get home or to a space with other people. These are systems that have evolved over hundreds of thousands of years to keep us alive—this is your survival instinct.

However, our ANS is not skilled at moderation. It hasn't adapted to a lifestyle filled with minor stressors, many of which are not life-threatening. For many of us, when we get called into our boss's office, fight with a loved one, or get stuck in traffic, this can set off our fight or flight mode, even though the stressful situation is not life-threatening. Our sympathetic nervous system can act as an alarm clock going off at random intervals throughout the day without an easy "off" switch to get back to homeostasis, a state of balance that allows the rest and digest system to become active.

The effect the sympathetic nervous system has on your body is as follows:

- Your heart rate increases.
- Your muscles tense.
- Digestion slows down.
- Your breath becomes shallow.
- Your palms begin to sweat.

If you've ever gotten butterflies in your stomach before doing something you were nervous about, you've experienced the effects of the sympathetic nervous system. If you pay attention to your body in the evening, you may notice some of these symptoms are present before bed.

If you can activate the deep rest of the parasympathetic nervous system, you'll notice that:

- Digestions improves.
- Your muscles relax.
- Your heart rate slows down.
- You can breathe deeper.

To sleep deeply, we need to be able to activate our PNS. However, switching off fight or flight mode is easier said than done. Yoga and meditation are two things that, when done regularly, help people get back to homeostasis quicker than those who don't meditate or practice yoga. We live in a world that is filled with distractions and technology designed to arouse our systems—doing activities that help you slip away from technology, job stress, and other worries, even if for a short time, can help to balance the nervous system.

The stress to your nervous system may not be something you are consciously aware of. I always thought that I was a calm and relaxed person, not quick to anger or easily flustered. Yet even things out of your control, like loud noises, traffic, or strong scents, can set off your SNS. I also had anxious thoughts about the future, which most of my peers had as well, but these thoughts affected me more strongly. One way to see how subtle stressors can be to activate our nervous system is by trying this short exercise:

Start by placing the butt of each palm on your eyebrows. Use your palms to pull your eyebrows up, causing your eyes to open wide. Stay here for a few moments, noticing your levels of alertness and any other sensations you're feeling.

Next, pull the eyebrows back down, causing your eyes to close. Stay here for a few moments and notice your alertness levels again.

For many people, just doing this exercise for two minutes can affect their level of arousal. We don't need strong medications to relax. We just need to use the tools that we already have to calm the nervous system.

How to improve sleep

It's not difficult to see why the parasympathetic nervous system is so important to sleep. To fall asleep, we need to relax our muscles, breathe deeply, and slow down our heart rates. While medication can help you fall asleep and stay asleep through the night, no medication can mimic the quality of sleep that your brain naturally creates. Taking medication (or alcohol or marijuana) is closer to what you'd experience from passing out, rather than experiencing a full sleep cycle.

Relaxation tools like yoga, meditation, and breathing exercises can help you to balance the nervous system so that you have more energy during the day and sleep better at night.[xxxv] Looking at your diet and other lifestyle factors, such as work, exercise, and home life, can also provide clues into what may be keeping you awake at night.

The goal of yoga or meditation isn't to stay relaxed all the time. If you're out for a walk with a friend and they trip and break their leg, you should go into fight or flight mode so that you can use all your energy to get them out of this situation safely. If walking in your neighborhood, it might be as simple as calling a taxi to bring you to the hospital. If you were out walking in the mountains on a hiking trip, this might involve physically supporting your friend down the mountain. To get the strength and energy to do this, you might need your body to go into fight or flight mode until you get your friend to safety.

The goal with yoga is to be able to switch between the systems as needed. In our example with your friend on a hiking trip, in an ideal situation, once you get your friend to safety, your system would begin to rebalance, and you'd be able to get into rest and digest mode within a few hours. However, some people can spend many hours or several days with a heightened nervous system after a stressful event, even if the danger has long passed, and even if the threat was minimal or non-life-threatening.

While Western medicine is fantastic at curing acute, temporary health challenges, for an issue as broad as sleep, I believe that a complementary or holistic approach is necessary. Note that I call this complementary and not alternative, as I think that we should use all of the tools at our disposal to improve our sleep and our health.

Relying solely on medication, which aims to treat symptoms over causes in many cases, can result in drug dependency. I wish that my doctor had used complementary medicine rather than just cycling me through different sleeping pills. Without getting to the root of what was causing my poor sleep, I only built resistance to the medication, and one after the other they all stopped working. It wasn't until I learned to balance my nervous system and quiet my mind that I was able to sleep well consistently. Further, yoga can have some of the same effects on your brain as medication, but without any harmful side effects. For example, several studies have shown that yoga decreases cortisol and other stress hormones in the brain.[xxxvi] Some yogic practices have also been found to increase melatonin.[xxxvii] Melatonin is a hormone that helps regulate sleep and is affected by light (that's why in Ayurveda you're meant to go to sleep and wake up with the sun, but more on that later). Due to artificial light and screens (phones, computers, TV, *etc.*), many people with insomnia have trouble producing melatonin at night. Yoga is one potential avenue to increase melatonin production in the evening drug-free.

My experiences getting treatment for sleep started over ten years ago, and in that time, I've witnessed healthcare regimens starting to change. Doctors are beginning to become aware of complementary forms of medicine and are beginning to recommend things like meditation, yoga, and other mindful and holistic treatments to patients suffering from chronic conditions. This shift is due to research studies that have shown that meditation and yoga can help people suffering from insomnia.

It's inspiring to see the healthcare system starting to move in the direction of holistic care, and recognizing the effect that our environments, thought patterns, diets, and nervous systems have on every aspect of our health. When looking at what is recommended by doctors, it's important to remember that sometimes politics and luck have more influence on what has become accepted "scientific" practice and what is considered "alternative" medicine.

So use your judgment and critical thinking when discussing treatment with your doctor. It's also essential to find a doctor who understands your challenges with sleep, takes them seriously, and is willing to explore a combination of different avenues to support you in getting the best night's sleep possible.

Action steps

1) It's time to become a "sleep detective!" Start a journal or create a spreadsheet to track your progress over the next two to three months. Write down your current evening and morning routines, what you do during the day, and what you're eating and drinking (especially in the late afternoon and evening).

2) If any stressful events happen, write them down. In the morning, record how you slept the night before, including how long it took you to fall asleep, if you woke up during the night, and how you felt in the morning.

3) At the end of each week, assess what you've written down in your journal and see if you can make any connections between your diet, activities, stress levels, and quality of sleep.

Step 2: The Yogic View of Sleep

Starting around age thirteen, falling asleep was never an easy feat for me. I would try to get into bed at a reasonable time, but I would toss and turn for hours. Often I would get up and do schoolwork (which I now know wasn't the best idea) or read a book (always a good idea) until I would fall asleep around three in the morning. Once I fell asleep, I would often wake up several times during the night, and I never felt refreshed in the morning. No matter what I tried in the evenings (chamomile tea, melatonin, odd-tasting magnesium supplements), I couldn't get to sleep before three a.m., and I couldn't sleep through the night.

When I started doing yoga, I would always feel relaxed after class, but at first, this wasn't translating into falling asleep that night. I would do yoga sporadically, when I had half an hour to watch the DVD I had bought or when a friend dragged me to her yoga studio. I never did the meditations or breathing exercises because I only thought of yoga as physical exertion, and I knew nothing about the medical benefits of yoga or mindfulness.

A few months later, when I signed up for the mindfulness-based stress reduction (MBSR) course, some of my homework was to meditate or do yoga every day. I started learning more about mindfulness and yoga and began applying what I was learning not only to my daily yoga and meditation sessions but to all aspects of my life. When I was stressed with work or school, I would close my door and do a short ten-minute meditation. If I was feeling overwhelmed in a social situation, I'd focus on my breath, coming back to the present moment, rather than letting my mind run wild with anxious thoughts. I was still struggling with sleep, but I noticed that I had more good nights than I had had before starting the course, and I felt both more relaxed and more energized during the day.

Then it happened—I fell asleep in a yoga class. I had heard of this phenomenon from teachers, but I had never come close to falling asleep in a yoga class. But one day in savasana, I felt myself slowly drifting off and then had to be shaken awake by the teacher at the end of the class.

Now that I'm a yoga teacher, I know that falling asleep during savasana is a somewhat regular occurrence. At least once a week, I'm gently rousing a slightly red-faced student from sleep at the end of the class. Yet, at the time, it felt revolutionary. I had scoffed at the idea of trying yoga or meditation when medication couldn't help me, yet here I was, at the end of an hour of stretching and holding odd poses, and I'd achieved more than any doctor had helped me achieve—I'd fallen asleep. I'd fallen asleep without taking drugs, without having any medical procedures, and without having someone hook electrodes up to my head. What I now know is that yoga helped me balance my nervous system, which allowed me to finally fall asleep.

Understanding yoga as medicine

In the West, we think of health as an absence of pain or symptoms. If you're able to function "normally" in society (*e.g.*, go to school or work full time, raise a family, *etc.*) we're often happy to suppress minor health issues with over-the-counter medications or just ignore them. This can lead health problems to go unchecked for many years. By aiming to have an absence of symptoms, rather than the full functioning of all of our systems, our health can slowly deteriorate until we are diagnosed with a chronic or life-threatening illness.

Yoga doesn't look at health as an absence of symptoms, but as the full functioning of all the systems in the body: physical, neurological, psychological, and emotional. Further, in yoga, these systems are not seen as separate entities we need to manage, but one interconnected system that balances body, mind, and spirit. If one of the systems is off, none of the other systems will be functioning at full capacity. If you've ever had a child who woke up with a stomachache and lowered appetite every morning before learning they were being made fun of at school, you've witnessed how all of these systems work together.

Many people see yoga as a series of complicated and awkward poses, often done by young, fit, and thin people. But yoga is more than just the physical postures. It is a medical system that includes poses, breathing exercises, meditation, diet, lifestyle changes, and more. It comes from the scientific tradition of Ayurveda, which is an ancient medical system focused on direct observation and turning inward. You may notice that once you start practicing yoga frequently, you are more aware of your symptoms and what is going on within your body not only at bedtime but throughout the day. This can help you better understand what is contributing to your insomnia, as well as any other health problems you may be having.

Yoga is such a powerful tool because, unlike medications, the power of yoga in healing becomes stronger over time.

The potent sleeping pills I was on all stopped working eventually because my body built up a resistance to the medication. It was not a viable long-term solution to my insomnia. However, yoga is a tool that continues to improve my sleep and overall health the longer I continue my practice. Each time you practice yoga, you help create and solidify new neural pathways that will help you balance the nervous system, reduce stress, increase resilience, boost your energy, and improve your sleep.

People often ask me how long it takes to see a benefit from yoga. The answer is: it depends. But I do know those that commit to a long-term regular practice see the best results. For this book, I am going to ask you to commit to eight weeks of a yoga and meditation practice. Committing to two months of a regular yoga practice (several times per week) should give you a taste of the power that yoga has over your sleep.

Each session only needs to be ten to fifteen minutes long. Consistency is more important than the length of time spent practicing. You also can banish ideas from your mind of super young, thin, fit yogis doing complicated poses. It is often the subtle movements and breathing exercises that can help us most. The practices in this book are suitable for most levels of strength, flexibility, endurance, and ability.

Insomnia according to Ayurveda

Ayurveda is the science of yoga. It's a Sanskrit word that translates roughly as "the science of life." This medical system has been practiced for over five thousand years on the Indian subcontinent and is still practiced in Ayurvedic hospitals and clinics throughout India today. While many in the West are exposed to yoga through yoga or fitness studios, yoga and meditation were often prescribed as part of a treatment plan by

Ayurvedic doctors.

Ayurveda is a medical system that looks at health complaints as part of a whole system, including the person's genetic disposition, environment, lifestyle habits, diet, and thought patterns. Ayurvedic practitioners use something called a dosha to help better understand the needs of their clients. A dosha is a genetic predisposition that can affect your physical characteristics, habits, and thought patterns. By understanding someone's dosha, Ayurvedic practitioners can better identify the root cause of the person's suffering and prescribe lifestyle changes to help resolve the problem.

The three doshas are:

- Kapha: Content and deliberate, Kaphas have a wide, sturdy build, thick hair, smooth skin, and tend to move slowly. Kaphas will be drawn to slow types of movement like yin yoga and enjoy nurturing those around them.
- Pitta: Fiery and intense, Pittas are quick to anger and often have a medium build with yellowish or reddish skin and are prone to red hair and freckles. Pittas are competitive and will be drawn to an active yoga practice like Ashtanga.
- Vata: Airy and scattered, Vatas love talking about many ideas and can never seem to get warm. They have a thin build often with knobbly joints. Vatas resist forming a routine and are drawn to quick movements like a vinyasa class.

Most people are primarily one or two doshas. The goal is to be able to balance these doshas so that none are over or underactive. According to Ayurveda, insomnia is the result of an overactive Vata dosha.

When a person's Vata is balanced, they're creative, quick-witted, and move quickly. However, when Vata is in excess, they might find their skin, nails, and hair are dry. Many Vatas experience problems with digestion and constipation, and their joints can get crackly and creaky. Most importantly, insomnia is a featured characteristic of Vata imbalance. A study from 2015 found that people who identified as Vata took longer to fall asleep and felt less rested in the morning.[xxxviii]

Vata imbalance can be caused by several things, such as lack of routine, moving homes, switching jobs, eating cold foods or living in a cold climate, poor diet, and stress. Since Ayurveda focuses on all the systems, not one, there is likely no singular cause for a Vata imbalance. However, once we know that Vata is out of whack, there are steps we can take to bring it back into balance, which will, in turn, improve your sleep.

Eating warm foods, creating a daily routine as well as morning and evening routines, doing grounding exercises, and practicing meditation can all help bring Vata into balance. We'll be discussing various techniques throughout this book that can help bring your Vata dosha back to a balanced state.

You may have noticed that many of the symptoms of Vata excess are similar to hyperarousal in the sympathetic nervous system. You can use whichever framing makes more sense to you; the therapy options we'll go over in this book are the same.

How yoga can help with insomnia and overall health

The wellness industry has become a multi-billion-dollar industry. What seemed like simple advice a couple of decades ago—eat more fruits and vegetables, exercise, don't smoke, don't drink in excess—has become complicated. Health is now sold in packages: in health food stores, at the supermarket, online, and at health clubs. If we want to be healthier, we should buy more "healthy" things. Even if that box of organic quinoa cookies is filled with sugar, or if the frozen meal with vegetables doesn't have the same nutrient density as a fresh meal, we have to pay a literal price for our health (not to mention that healthy food is often more expensive and more time-intensive to prepare than its fast and processed counterparts). With so many conflicting messages and so much politics involved (don't even get me started on those green health checks), it can be hard to know what changes we should be making in our lives.

Yoga is such a powerful tool for this because it is based on observation of oneself. When you develop a yoga practice, you'll start to notice how you feel after eating certain foods. You'll see if you feel more aroused after doing a particular activity and thus know not to do it in the evening close to bedtime. You'll be aware of the forces in your life that are draining your energy versus the ones that are giving you energy. Once you begin to build self-awareness, you'll be less reliant on a medical authority to tell you what to do to be healthy and more in tune to the specific needs of your own body.

What's more, we all know that eating healthier, exercising more, and turning off the TV before bed would help us feel better. It can be challenging to make these changes. Packaged fast foods are available at every corner, and you don't always have the time to cook a fresh meal. We live in a culture where being busy is more valued than being happy (or sleeping, which, in my opinion, is closely tied to happiness). Further, breaking patterns and committing to a new routine, no matter how much you think it will help you, is difficult.

Yoga can help you make the changes that you want to make in your life. It can help you make better decisions, break patterns, and create new, healthier routines that will nourish you. When you're aware of the toll your actions and choices make on your body, you'll be better able to make the day-to-day changes. When you're living mindfully, you'll know that much as you want that sugary candy bar, you don't need it. When you're able to commit to a challenging yoga pose or moment in meditation, you'll be ready to take on other challenges in your day.

In yoga, creating a new routine or mental groove is called

samskara. The same idea in Western medicine is called neuroplasticity. We used to believe that our brains start developing at birth and stop around twenty-six or twenty-seven. However, in the past few years, research has shown that our brains are more malleable than we think. Making changes to our brain structure is possible well into adulthood.[xxxix] One thing that can affect brain structure and functioning is meditation.[xl] In yoga, we create new grooves (or samskaras) in the brain by doing something over and over. This could be a sound, the breath, or a movement. By committing to a yoga and meditation practice daily (or several times a week), you'll begin to create a new groove in your brain. These changes can make it easier to switch on your relaxation response, help you fall asleep faster and have a higher quality of sleep, and create more gray matter in the hippocampus, which is the part of the brain associated with learning and memory.[xli]

The yogic toolbox

There are many tools in yoga besides the physical postures that can help improve sleep, balance the nervous system, and create a healthy body, mind, and spirit. You may want to experiment with different yogic tools to see which best fit into your life, and which have the greatest benefit to you. Yoga is an experiential medicine, so I recommend choosing one to two more tools in addition to postures and breathing to start with. Record your observations and continue with your sleuthing work by trying different things!

The essentials of yoga therapy

Asana: Physical postures. This is what most of us in the West think of when we think of yoga. Whether you practice at home, in a studio, or with a private teacher, there will likely be at least some asana in your practice. This can be more difficult strength-building postures, or it can be subtle movements of the body designed to restore or activate the nervous system.

Pranayama: Breathing exercises. Breath is essential to a yoga practice and is often linked to the asanas you do in a class, as well as included as its own exercise at the beginning and end of practice. The breath is a powerful tool for balancing the nervous system. Pranayama should always be incorporated into asana practice, but it can also be practiced on its own.

Other yogic tools

Pratyahara: Drawing inward. This refers to bringing your attention, focus, and energy to your inner life. Instead of focusing on what is going on around you (sounds, sights, smells, *etc.*), you focus entirely on the inner sensations of your body and mind. This is usually practiced in meditation.

Dhyana: Meditation. Breathing, drawing inward, and concentration are all of the aspects that lead to meditation. However, according to the ancient yogis, meditation referred to closing off thoughts as well as outward sensations. While it's impossible to turn your thoughts off completely, aiming to lessen the frequency and intensity of our thoughts through drawing inward, concentrating, and engaging in breathing exercises is what the yogis refer to as meditation. It is said that when you can completely shut off thoughts, you will reach samadhi, or enlightenment.

Diet: A vital part of Ayurveda and most health systems, finding a diet that works for you can be integral to balancing the nervous system and helping the body function at full capacity. This book includes tips on an Ayurvedic Vata-pacifying diet in Step 7.

Oils: Ayurvedic practitioners often prescribe oils for massage or incense burning that can help calm Vata and prepare the body for sleep.

Cleansing: Cleansing techniques such as the neti pot or other breathing exercises can be used to keep the body functioning well.

Karma Yoga: In the West, we'd call this community service. Feeling connected to a community and being able to donate your time and effort to a cause that you care about can be a great way to boost healthy feelings and give back to your community.

Faith: While yoga is based in Hinduism, any faith in a religion or higher power can be used as a tool for spiritual healing (though belief in a deity is not necessary!).

In this book, we'll explore different yoga techniques and exercises, and you'll be able to select the tools that make the most sense for your life and your health.

Action steps

1) Take this dosha quiz and this vikriti quiz to discover what your dosha is and if you currently have an imbalance (quizzes can be found on www.yogainternational.com).

2) Write down your thoughts about your dosha. Do you identify with the physical and psychological traits of your primary dosha or doshas?

3) Build your yoga toolbox. Write down the different yogic tools you would like to try for sleep. Then circle the ones you'd like to implement in the first two weeks.

4) Analyze your sleep journal after one week. Do you see any patterns? Observe for another week before making any significant changes, so you know what baseline you're starting with, but make notes for any patterns or interesting observations you see!

Step 3: Creating a Healthy Sleep Environment

I've been lucky enough to have traveled and lived in many different places around the world over the past seven years. During this time, I've seen how much location and environment can affect my sleep patterns, my mood, and my energy levels. When I lived in an ashram in India, I was up at four thirty every morning and went to sleep at nine at night. When I was in the humid rainforest of Peru, it was normal for me to wake up around eight in the morning, have an hour-long nap in the afternoon, and be asleep again by midnight. I've also seen how hard it is to fall asleep in a noisy apartment on an ambulance route in central London. Or how even though I often fall asleep on long flights or train rides, I never wake up feeling quite as refreshed as if I was in my bed.

You may have noticed this in your life, too. If you fall

asleep in the car or on the couch in front of the TV, you won't feel as rested when you wake up as if you were fully reclined in bed. Also, you may notice that if you stay in a hotel or with a friend for a night, you don't sleep as well as you did at home. This is because it can be harder to fall asleep in unknown environments, and we get the best rest when we are fully (or almost fully) reclined.

The environment that we sleep in, while not a cure for insomnia, can have a significant impact on the quality of our sleep.

When my insomnia first started, I often stayed up all night reading the newest Harry Potter book or watching television. Instead of helping, this only made my insomnia worse as I lay in bed, trying to fall asleep to the dulcet tones of Late Night with Conan O'Brien. I told myself at least I was getting a good laugh before I would have to drag my sleep-deprived brain out of bed in the mornings, yet this strategy was not conducive to good sleep.

One contributing factor of this onset of insomnia could have been my age. Teenagers have a later circadian rhythm than older adults or younger kids and will naturally feel sleepy a few hours later than those groups. Many sleep experts think we should push school times for high school and university back a couple of hours. The primary pushback is often stereotypes about teenagers just being lazy or wanting to party, as well as consideration for the working hours of the teachers. Often, the only way I could drift off was by having the television or music on in the background.[2] I eventually shifted completely to music (and now sometimes use audiobooks), as I now understand how harmful the light from the television can be for sleep.

While it's essential to use the other tools in this book, making small changes to your environment can help you sleep better immediately. Also, we want to make sure that we are doing

---

2. Putting on my sleep detective hat, this was a clear sign that an overactive mind was one of the leading causes of my insomnia.

all the things we can control to create the right environment for sleep. This will help us better measure the effects of the yoga and meditation exercises I'll go over in this book.

When doing scientific research, scientists have to control for as many variables as possible. For example, if we decided to see if yoga helped people sleep and divided them into two groups, one group who did yoga and one who did not, and then tried to measure the results, we wouldn't get a lot of valuable information from this experiment. To get value, we'd need to know how each participant slept before, what their diet was like during the trial, the environments they were sleeping in, their age, and whether or not they had kids, partners, or pets that might get into bed with them. Without controlling for this other information, it would be almost impossible to tell what effects the yoga was having and what was just chance or influenced by other factors.

So, to best see what lifestyle changes are working for us, we want to create the most neutral and scientifically backed environment possible. Then we can see how yoga and meditation affect our nightly habits.

When my doctors recommended that I use good "sleep hygiene," I was skeptical for many of the reasons I was skeptical of yoga. It was nearly impossible for me to fall asleep at a reasonable hour. Getting blackout curtains or a white noise machine wasn't going to help that. I felt like they weren't taking my health issues seriously, or worse yet, that they were blaming me for my insomnia.

Now that my understanding of health and sleep has changed, I can see how important it is to create both the right physical and psychological environment for sleep. Here are my best tips for creating the right environment for sleep:

Mental relaxation

- Take a bath or shower. Warm water can be therapeutic, relaxing your mind and sore muscles. Also, after you get out of a warm bath, your body temperature will slowly cool, mimicking what happens to your body temperature when you fall asleep. Research shows that people who take a warm bath or shower before bed fall asleep quicker and have a deeper sleep than those who don't.[xlii]

- Keep your room cool or use a fan (at least in the summer months). Our body temperature needs to drop to fall into a deep sleep. While you don't want to be uncomfortably cold, using a fan or sticking your feet out of the bottom of the blanket can help regulate your temperature for bedtime.

- Finish any work/studying/chores at least two hours before bedtime.

- Drink an herbal tea such as mint, chamomile, lavender, or valerian root.[3]

- Do a relaxing activity such as reading a book, listening to an audiobook, listening to music, or talking with your partner. Avoid looking at electronics and avoid doing anything stimulating. For example, now is not the time to read an action-packed book or listen to rock music. Choose music and books that won't make your heart race.

- Reduce as much noise as you can before bed. If you live in a noisy area, consider getting noise-canceling headphones or earplugs to help you sleep. A white noise machine or a machine that creates nature noises can also help counter the effects of a noisy neighborhood.

------

3. Valerian root can be a powerful sleeping herb. While gentler than most sleep medications, this should still be used sparingly for when you really need help to get to sleep, as it can cause addiction.

- Do a restorative yoga practice in the evening (see Step 6) or meditate before bed. Both can help relax the nervous system.
- If you aren't scent-free, some scents through incense or essential oils can help induce relaxation. Some to try are jasmine, lavender, vanilla, rose, or anything you find pleasing and calming.
- If you have pets, don't allow them to sleep in the bed with you. Snoring, noises, and movement from bed partners can all interrupt sleep. While it's unlikely you'll want to send your human partner to the spare bedroom, keeping pets in a separate space at night can aid sleep.

Darkness

Before the electric lightbulb, most people would go to bed a couple of hours after sunset and wake just before or around sunrise. After sunset, it was impossible to continue doing work, and people had to engage in relaxing evening activities. Now that technology has surpassed the need for daylight to be productive, it's easy for people to stay up late working, studying, or watching television. When we expose ourselves to artificial lighting, we are tricking our bodies into thinking it is still daytime, and thus delaying the creation of melatonin and other hormones that signal to the brain it's time for sleep. While it's probably unrealistic for most people nowadays to sleep and wake with the sun, we can try to honor this connection by creating darkness when preparing for sleep. If you do need to check your phone or computer, set your electronics to "night mode" to reduce the amount of blue light you're taking in. When it comes time for bed:

- Check to make sure there are no electronics on in your room, and even clocks should be covered or turned away.

- Try to keep your room as dark as possible. If you live in a bright area or big city, it might be worth investing in blackout curtains.
- If your room is still bright or your partner needs a light on, consider using an eye mask to create darkness.
- When you wake up in the morning, try to get natural light as soon as possible by opening the windows, sitting outside, or going for a walk.

Bed

Ensuring that your mattress and pillows are comfortable, your sheets are clean, and there's nothing in your room you're allergic to can all help you get a better night's sleep. If your mattress is uncomfortable, it can be a big investment to replace, but remember that sleeping better can add years to your life and help you overcome and prevent illness, so it is a long-term investment that will more than pay off.

Diet

While eating food that is nourishing for your body is essential for good health, there are a few specific foods that can inhibit or support sleep. Here are some of the most popular foods that can hinder sleep and should be avoided at any point in the afternoon, if not all day:

- Caffeine. Caffeine is found in coffee, tea (except for herbal tea), chocolate, dark sodas, other snacks, and some medications. If you're taking medication in the evening or eating packaged foods, read the labels carefully so that you're not consuming caffeine in the evening. The half-life of caffeine is five to seven hours. However, after that five to seven hours, you'll still have fifty percent of the caffeine in your system, which is quite a lot! Not only does caffeine make it harder to fall asleep, but it can also halve your amount of deep, slow-wave sleep and make it more likely for you to wake during the night.

- Coffee or black tea should only be drunk before noon. If your insomnia is severe, you may want to cut caffeine out completely.

- Decaf coffee is a decent alternative for those who love the taste, but decaf coffee still has fifteen to thirty percent of the caffeine content of regular coffee, so even it should be avoided after two p.m. (same for beverages with mild amounts of caffeine like green tea). Caffeine blocks sleepy chemicals in the brain, so it tricks you into thinking you're awake, but it doesn't give you more energy. This can be dangerous for insomniacs or those with illnesses like chronic fatigue because it can mask your symptoms but is not a long-term solution. Avoiding or severely limiting caffeine can improve your sleep dramatically. Age also makes you more sensitive to caffeine, so if you drank it no problem when you were younger but are having trouble sleeping now, it might be worth cutting it out.

- Alcohol. Taking a "nightcap" is common wisdom for helping people fall asleep, but consuming alcohol can make your sleep worse. Booze can often help you fall asleep, but the quality of your sleep will usually be worse, and you are more likely to wake up during the night. Having one drink in the evening should be okay, but if you have more than a couple in the evening or make it a regular habit, expect to wake up in the night when you sober up or need to go to the bathroom. Also, alcohol is more likely to produce a deep sleep that more resembles passing out than the healthy five-stage sleep cycle.

- Sugar. New research has shown that sugar can negatively affect your sleep.[xliii] What's frustrating is that poor sleep can lead to sugar cravings, in turn making you sleep worse at night and then making you crave sugar more the next day. If you have a sweet tooth, it would be wise to limit your sugar intake throughout the day, sticking to fruit and cutting out juices or artificial sugars. Perhaps you could plan one to two days per week where you're allowed your favorite sugary treat, but try to limit your sugar intake to natural sugars most of the time.

- Supplements. Some supplements (magnesium, valerian root) or herbal teas (chamomile, lavender)[xliv] can help you fall asleep faster and sleep more deeply. Using supplements like these is far better than using prescription sleep medication and can make a nice addition to your bedtime routine, but ideally, we should be working toward sleeping naturally without any aids, as that will provide the highest quality of sleep.

Creating routine

Creating a routine is a crucial sleep aid, according to both Western and Ayurvedic medicine. In Ayurveda, creating a routine is one of the most helpful things we can do to calm Vata. Vatas by nature reject habit and often like living creatively and spontaneously. However, creating a routine can be very beneficial for improving the health and creativity of those with a Vata imbalance. Sleep researchers also promote creating a routine to fall asleep and wake up at the same time each night. Many people will try to wake up early during the week and sleep in on the weekends, but this is not a good long-term strategy because we can't make up for lost time when it comes to sleep—especially not over a two-day weekend.

It's not clear precisely how much sleep we need each night for optimal health. In part, we don't know because it varies from individual to individual. However, most research shows that we require a minimum of eight hours of sleep, and possibly as much as ten or eleven hours—especially if you are recovering from illness.

These hours don't all need to be at night. Taking an afternoon nap can be an effective way to get one to two more hours of sleep in if you're a short sleeper. But if you get less than seven or eight hours of sleep in a twenty-four-hour period, you will begin to suffer from sleep deprivation. Many people who are busy with jobs and families sleep less during the week in the hopes to make it up over the weekend or when on holiday. Routine can help us get the same amount of sleep each night so that we're not cutting sleep time in hopes of making up for it the next day.

Creating routine is about more than setting regular sleep and wake up times. Having relaxing activities to do in the evening and rousing activities to do in the morning can help ease your body through the transitions of sleeping and waking. Creating a routine may take some experimentation. I can make recommendations on what works for my students and me, but each person is different and will respond to different activities. Begin by choosing two or three activities that resonate with you, and record how you feel each morning and evening after your routine. After a few weeks, assess which activities you'd like to keep, which you'd like to remove, and which you'd like to add.

Before creating your routine, I have one more note about sleep and wake up times. In university, I had a roommate who was up at seven or eight every morning. While I had to sometimes wake up at this time to get to work, I was not "awake." I would lie in bed, checking my emails or reading a book, begrudgingly getting up at the last minute to pull on some clothes, leaving myself no buffer to get to work on time. In contrast, my roommate was cheery, conversational, well-dressed, and often had time to do her hair and makeup before leaving.

You've probably seen examples of this in your own life too. Some people are energetic in the morning, and then after dinner start to calm down. When I was ready to start gabbing and making jokes at nine or ten, my roommate was already getting ready for bed, sometimes nodding off during conversation. Some people, like me, are slow to get moving in the morning and have more energy in the afternoon and evening. In the sleep world, we call the early risers "larks" and the late risers "owls." Everyone has a different sleep rhythm, and it will vary by several hours from person to person. On average, this difference is usually only a couple hours between larks and owls. There may be an evolutionary purpose for this: staggering sleep times amongst tribe members would make it easier to set watch times without anyone falling asleep during their shift. Instead of trying to fight your natural rhythm of sleepiness and wakefulness, see if you can build your morning, evening, and daily routines to accommodate your ideal sleep schedule. Unfortunately, as a society, we tend to favor larks over owls. Depending on the kind of work you do, you may have a hard time convincing your boss to let you work ten to six instead of nine to five or eight to four. But if it's possible to make tweaks to your schedule to follow your natural flow of energy, all the better.

Evening routine

When creating an evening routine, I like to work backward. What time do you want to wake up in the morning? What time would you need to be sleeping by to get at least eight hours of sleep? For example, let's say you want to wake up at seven a.m. This means going to sleep no later than eleven p.m. Below I've included a routine with sample activities based on my bedtime and morning routines. You can take this routine to start with and adapt it to fit with your interests and lifestyle.

7:00 p.m.: dinner

7:30 p.m.: watching TV, reading, spending time with

friends or family

9:00 p.m.: warm bath or shower

9:30 p.m.: making a warm herbal tea (chamomile, jasmine, or similar sleep-promoting tea), reading a book, or listening to soothing music—nothing too stimulating like fast music or an action-packed novel.

10:00 p.m.: preparing for bed, getting into pyjamas, making the bed, dimming the lights, *etc.*

10:30 p.m.: in bed with the lights out (potential to listen to an audiobook, music, or a podcast if that helps you sleep)

11:00 p.m.: sleep

Morning routine

Creating a morning routine with things that excite you can help you be more alert for the rest of the day. If you have trouble getting up in the morning, knowing that you have this routine rather than having to head straight to work or other obligations can help make getting out of bed less painful. If, like me, you're an owl and struggle to get moving in the morning, it can help to plan something you enjoy first thing in the morning. It could be watching the next episode in your current television series, reading a book, eating your favorite breakfast, or going for a walk outside. Here's an example of a morning routine that you can use to create your own:

7:00 a.m.: wake up

7:10 a.m.: fifteen- to twenty-minute meditation or gentle yoga practice

7:30 a.m.: making tea, journaling, reading, going for a walk outside

8:00 a.m.: breakfast

8:30 a.m.: ready to start the day!

It can also help to use your bed and bedroom only for sleep. This is a rule I am terrible at following since I work from home and sometimes enjoy working from bed, especially in the morning, but I try to abide by this rule most of the time. If you have an illness that leaves you fatigued during the day, it can be a good idea to set up a sofa or bed in another area of the house so that your bedroom is reserved only for sleeping at night. I recently visited Frida Kahlo's house in Mexico City. Frida was plagued by multiple illnesses and injuries that left her in pain and severely disabled. In her house she had a daytime bed which she would use to rest in during the day (and sometimes paint from!). At night, she would retire to her bedroom, where she would sleep for the night.

Another tool you might choose to incorporate into your day is napping. This won't be possible for people working a nine-to-five job (unless you live in a region where taking an afternoon nap is the norm, such as Mediterranean Europe or Latin America). But if you have a flexible schedule, taking a short nap around one or two in the afternoon can be beneficial in supplementing your nighttime sleep, especially if you've gotten less than eight hours. If you often notice yourself getting tired in the early afternoon, this might be a helpful tool with which to experiment.

It will take some experimentation to find what works for you, but by using these tips and the yoga and meditation practices we'll cover in the next three chapters, I'm sure you'll be able to create a routine that helps you sleep better and works for your lifestyle!

Be strict with your routine when you are first getting started and trying to figure out what works best for you. However, one of the biggest stress-busters is joy. So if you'd occasionally like to throw your routine out the window to go out with friends or stay up late reading a book or watching a movie, by all means, go for it and enjoy every moment. Just don't allow it to become a regular habit, as it's hard to find joy when you aren't sleeping well.

Action steps

1) Write down which sleep hygiene tips you'd like to implement. Create a step-by-step list of how and when you will do each one.
2) Write down your ideal morning and evening routines. How different are they from your current morning and evening habits? If they're very different, circle the parts that will be easiest to implement and start with those for a couple of weeks!

Step 4: Meditations for Better Sleep

Once I went to see a behavioural therapist, and she suggested I do a deep breathing exercise at night. She told me that when I couldn't sleep, I should count my breaths up to ten, then back down to one, and that I should imagine being on the beach or by the ocean while I was doing this. At the time, I thought this was a silly idea. If strong medication wasn't helping me, how would deep breathing and thinking of the beach help me? Surely she was mad. I think I tried the exercises for a night or two and felt more relaxed while I was doing them, but without immediate results, I didn't continue.

Then, several years later, I started the mindfulness-based stress reduction (MBSR) course. This time, I was committed to trying anything. I felt jaded by all the sleeping pills that had stopped working and was hoping there was something else that could help me get to sleep.

At first, I was skeptical of the meditations, but I had

285

committed to giving the course my full attention for eight weeks. During the first session, several people in the group fell asleep. While I felt more relaxed during the meditations, I wasn't one of the students who ended the meditation snoring.

I spoke with the course leader about my insomnia and about feeling more relaxed after the meditations. She recommended if I couldn't sleep, I should do the body scan in bed. I could also try some of the breathing exercises before bed to help me relax.

When I started meditating in bed, it didn't always result in my falling asleep afterward. But I always felt calmer and more rested after doing the meditations, almost as if I had had a little nap. As I started adding the other yoga and meditation exercises throughout the day, I realized I was falling asleep faster at night, or when I wasn't falling asleep, meditation could help me get there. I realized that breathing exercises, visualizations, and meditations could make changes to my nervous system and hormone levels and help me to fall asleep. Despite my skepticism when I was younger, my breath and my mind could be more powerful tools than even the most potent medications.

Further, I learned that the most effective path is not always the easiest path. It took more than just a few days for the effects of yoga and meditation to kick in. It's a process that continues to change and grow as I do and requires dedication, patience, and humility. By using the tools mindfulness and meditation provided me, I was able to get to a place where I felt in control of my health and my sleep habits.

What is mindfulness?

Practicing mindfulness, whether it's through meditation, yoga, or making mindful choices in our day-to-day lives, is an invaluable tool for balancing the autonomic nervous system. Mindfulness is being present in the moment. This means you're not thinking about what you want to make for dinner, the errand you need to run, or the awkward thing you said to your coworker. You are only thinking about what is going on in the present, which, in this case, is sitting or lying down in meditation. Mindfulness is a simple concept, but hard to put into practice. Our minds are constantly racing with a hundred different thoughts and ideas. Like most things, mindfulness takes practice. No one can shut their mind off completely, but you will find as you continue to practice these meditations you will get better at staying present.

Meditation is the perfect time to practice mindfulness, but we can practice mindfulness at any time. I believe that my yoga practice is made stronger the more present I am during my session. Beyond my yoga practice, whether I'm walking, eating, or spending time with friends, mindfulness has made me more aware of what my body needs to thrive.

Mindfulness meditations for sleep

Body Scan

The body scan is one of the first meditations I practiced regularly. It's a pillar of mindfulness meditation and is particularly helpful because it keeps you in the present moment while also giving you various things to focus on to stop your mind from wandering. Do know that if your mind does start to roam, this is very normal and happens to everyone! Take a moment to acknowledge where your mind has wandered to, then choose to bring your focus back to the meditation. This meditation is best done lying down on a yoga mat, but it can also be done sitting in a chair or lying down in bed.

How to do it:

- Lie down on a yoga mat or your bed. Begin by focusing on your breath, breathing slowly and deeply.
- As you inhale, bring your focus to your feet, noticing any sensations in your toes, heels, or the top or bottom of the feet. Hold your attention here for two or three breaths. On the next exhale, release your attention.
- On the next inhale, move the focus up to the ankles and calves.
- Suspend passing judgment on the things you notice in your body. Allow any feelings to reside in your body—just for the moment.
- Continue moving your attention through the body from your toes to your head, changing your focus every few breaths.

Breathing Meditation

As you can guess from the name, this meditation focuses on your breath. You can visualize your breath moving in and out of the body and through the respiratory system, focus on physical sensations of the breathing, or count your breaths to stay focused.

How to do it:
- Lie down or sit in a comfortable position free from distractions or interruptions.
- Begin by focusing on your breath. Notice how it moves in and out of your nose (or mouth).
- Notice how the breath feels moving in and out of your nostrils, all the way down into your diaphragm.
- Picture the breath moving into your nose, through your throat, through your lungs, and down into your belly. Imagine you can see the breath retracing this route back out into the air.

- After five to ten rounds of visualizing your breath, count your breaths up to ten, then back down to one, counting each breath on the exhale.
- Once you've come back to one, take a few more breaths, noticing how your body feels, and then open your eyes.

Yoga Nidra and Guided Visualizations

Yoga Nidra stems from the tantric school of yoga. As opposed to the mindfulness-based meditations which encourage observation of your thoughts as a third party, the tantric school encourages you to engage with and fully feel thoughts and emotions as they come through. This makes this type of meditation harder to practice on your own without a teacher or recording, as having a leader to guide you through the practice helps avoid getting consumed by thoughts or feelings. These meditations usually involve a guided journey where you can fully experience both your inner and outer surroundings. You can search for a yoga Nidra teacher in your area, or if you're interested in trying a recording, please send me an email at kayla@arogayoga.com, and I will send you a recorded session!

Mindful goal setting

If mindfulness means staying present in the moment, how can we plan for the future or work toward goals?

In yoga, instead of setting an outcome-based goal, such as "I want to fall asleep within thirty minutes tonight," we set goals that are effort-based. An effort-based goal might look like:

- I will meditate for fifteen minutes each day.
- I will practice yoga four times per week.
- I will cut out caffeine any time after lunch.

As you can see, mindful or yogic goal setting is based on the process, rather than the outcome. No matter how much we would like to, we cannot control the outcomes of our actions, but we can choose our actions. It's also important to remember that when we focus on nourishing activities such as meditation or eating well, the process can be just as important as the outcome. Even if you don't fall asleep after doing a meditation practice, the act of meditating on its own comes with a host of benefits for your body and mind, even if it wasn't the outcome that you hoped for on this particular occasion.

When setting goals for yourself, remember to keep yogic goal setting in mind. Focus on the factors that you can control and the actions that you can take, rather than the outcome, which is not something we can control.

Action steps

1) Write down any of the meditations from this chapter that you'd like to try.
2) Choose one and practice it for fifteen minutes three times this week.
3) Take a piece of paper or a page in your journal and write down mindful goals for everything we've covered in this book so far: creating an environment for good sleep, creating routine, and mindfulness meditation. Leave space to add in goals for the next three chapters!

Step 5: Breathing Exercises for Better Sleep

When I was sick with chronic fatigue syndrome, I started working with an occupational therapist to help me get more done with my limited energy. In one of our first sessions, he asked me if I practiced meditation. I told him I didn't. He asked me if I got stressed or overwhelmed with the work I had to do while I was sick. I told him I did. He then asked me to do this exercise:

- Make a fist with one hand, and take as many short, fast breaths as you can.
- Notice how easy or hard it was to keep your hand in a fist.
- Release your hand and stretch the fingers out.
- Now, make a fist again, but this time take a long, slow inhale, and an even longer exhale.

- Notice how easy or hard it was to keep your fist tight this time.

For most people, it's much easier to keep your muscles tight when you're breathing shallow and fast than when you're breathing deep and slow. So many of us hold pain and tension in our bodies and go to great lengths to try to relieve this pain or tension. That may involve seeing a massage therapist or physical therapist, taking medications, or working with a doctor. While some of these methods can certainly be helpful, they can also be expensive and ineffective. I was surprised to learn that a simple breathing exercise, in just two minutes, could have so much effect on muscular tension.

Muscular tension is critical to sleep because, as you may have guessed, it is hard to relax enough to drift into a dream state if you have tense muscles. If you notice a clenched jaw or restless leg at night, I believe these breathing exercises will be especially helpful for you in relaxing in the evening.

The mind-body connection

The mind-body (or body-mind) connection is the idea that all systems of the body are interconnected. According to Eastern medical traditions, the mind, body, and all the processes of the body are irrevocably linked. You may have heard the phrase "mind over matter," yet what is often missed is we can also use "matter over mind." For example, muscular tension is often a result of psychological stress. By focusing on reducing muscular tension, we can reduce the amount of psychological stress we are experiencing. At the same time, lowering our mental stress levels will lower tension in the body. This is why yoga focuses on balancing the entire system rather than just focusing on yoga poses or mindfulness techniques.

The breath is one of the best demonstrators of how our

systems are connected. In the body, we have automatic functions, such as your heartbeat, digestive system, circulation, *etc.*, as well as voluntary systems, which can be things like moving your muscles, chewing, swallowing, *etc.* The breath is the connector between these two systems. You can control your breathing to some extent. You can choose to slow down or speed up your breath, breathe deeply or shallowly, or even hold your breath for a time. However, you can't completely stop breathing. If you tried to hold your breath for too long, you'd pass out and start breathing again. In yoga, we aim to link all systems of the body and mind. The breath is a tangible link between the voluntary and involuntary systems of the body. Learning to use the control you have over your breath as a tool for healing can be a powerful way to relax in the evening and prepare for bedtime.

How to breathe well

Diaphragmatic breathing is essential to yogic breathwork. Diaphragmatic breathing is a breath that goes all the way into your belly (or, well, diaphragm), making your stomach rise as you inhale and go down as you exhale. To know if you're breathing well, try this short exercise:

- Lie on your back, placing one hand on your belly and one hand on your chest. Breathe normally.
- Notice where in your abdomen you're feeling the breath. Do you feel a rise in your chest that doesn't make it any lower? Or can you feel your stomach moving as you breathe?
- Does your stomach inflate as you inhale and deflate as you exhale? Or does the opposite happen? This is known as reverse breathing. While some believe that reverse breathing can have benefits such as increased lung capacity

and a boost in energy, breathing this way all the time can make it harder to relax at night.

If you notice that you are breathing only into your chest, or your breathing is reversed, take five to ten minutes a day to practice diaphragmatic breathing. Breathe slowly in through your nose and imagine that you are pulling the air down into your belly, then slowly let the air come back out, moving up to your chest, through your throat, and out through your nose. After you practice, notice how you feel. Eventually, this type of breathing will feel natural to you, and you won't have to think about it.

Using breath control to help us relax is one of the main limbs of a yogic practice. When doing breathing exercises, we are honoring the links between the automatic and voluntary systems of the body and extending this link to all of our systems. Breathing exercises can help balance the nervous system and also help clear your mind, as you'll be focusing on your breath rather than running thoughts. You can do these exercises just before bed or at any point when you feel you need to calm the nervous system.

Breathing exercises for insomnia

4-7-8 Breathe

This breathing exercise includes holding your breath and extending exhales, both breathing techniques that can help activate the parasympathetic nervous system. 4-7-8 is a great exercise to do just before getting in bed for the night, or when you are already in bed. It is one of the most powerful breathing exercises for falling asleep.

How to do it:
- Sit or lie down in bed in a comfortable position free from distractions.
- Inhale for four counts.

- Hold your breath for seven counts.
- Exhale for eight counts.
- If this is too much of a challenge, you can reduce it so that it is the 4-6-7 or 4-5-6 exercise. As you continue practicing breathing deeply, your lung capacity will expand, and you will be able to hold your breath for a longer time.
- Repeat for five to ten rounds or until you feel yourself starting to nod off to sleep.

Extended Exhales

A simplified version of the above exercise, extending your exhales is the perfect place to start for beginners, as it doesn't involve holding your breath. Holding your breath can be a powerful tool for relaxation, but if you're not used to it, it can sometimes cause stress. Lengthening your exhale is a great way to prepare the body for deep relaxation.

How to do it:
- Sit or lie down in a comfortable position free from distractions.
- Inhale for four counts.
- Exhale for six counts.
- Inhale for four counts.
- If it feels comfortable, extend the exhale to seven or eight counts.
- Continue for ten to fifteen rounds once you've found a comfortable exhaling length (up to double the length of the inhale).

Counting the Breath (like counting sheep, but better!)

This straightforward mindfulness breathing exercise can be done at any time of the day when you need to relax and refresh. If you've had a stressful evening or were watching TV or reading before bed, this exercise can help clear your mind and get your focus back on sleep. It's age-old wisdom to count things to fall asleep, and the real secret of the counting is that it helps your mind focus on something immediate, so your thoughts don't wander to other stresses. Counting the breath adds to the benefits because deep breathing is so beneficial to triggering your relaxation response!

How to do it:
- Lie in bed or sit in a comfortable position.
- Begin breathing deeply in and out of your belly. Notice what your breath feels like in the body and the rhythm of your breathing.
- Once you are comfortable, begin counting the breaths on each exhale. Continue until ten, and then count back down to one.
- Repeat this cycle four to five times or until you feel ready for bed.

Progressive Relaxation

This breathing exercise combines breathing with muscular movement to release muscular tension. If you have restless leg syndrome or notice a lot of tension in your body (like shoulders hunching or hips tightening) when you're in bed at night, this exercise may be helpful for you. I recommend practicing this sometime in the evening rather than directly before bed.

How to do it:
- Lie down in a comfortable position, perhaps using a support under your neck and knees.
- Begin by activating your deep belly breathing and focusing on the sensation of each inhale and exhale.

YOGA FOR CHRONIC ILLNESS

- When ready, on your next inhale, squeeze the muscles in your feet, toes, and ankles as hard as you can.
- On your exhale, release.
- Take a cleansing round of breath.
- On your next inhale, squeeze the muscles in your calves as hard as you can.
- On your exhale, release.
- After you've made your way through your entire body, take several deep, mindful breaths to finish the practice.

Ujayi Breath

Also known as "Darth Vader" breath, Ujayi breath is sometimes used during a yoga practice but can also be used as a pranayama practice on its own and can be very calming to the nervous system.

How to do it:

- Sit in a comfortable position on a chair or on the floor. This practice can also be done lying down.
- Inhale as usual, and as you exhale, make a "hhhhhhhh" sound with the back of your throat as if you are trying to fog up a mirror (or imitate Darth Vader).
- Continue making this noise on each exhale.
- Count up to ten and back down to one, doing as many rounds as you need to feel relaxed.

Action steps

1) Write down any of the meditations from this chapter that you'd like to try and add them to your goals sheet you made in the last chapter.
2) Choose one and practice it for fifteen minutes three times this week!

Step 6: Yoga Sequences for Better Sleep

A quick note before starting this chapter: you should speak with your doctor before starting any new physical activity plan. Your doctor can help you identify any potential areas of support that you'll want to discuss with your yoga therapist or be aware of when starting a home practice. The first rule of yoga is that we don't want to make anything worse. If you have bad knees, high or low blood pressure, or anything else that may affect your yoga practice, you should talk with your doctor to discuss if there are any postures you should avoid, or adapt, in your yoga practice. If you work with a qualified yoga therapist, they will be able to help you adapt the poses based on your doctor's recommendations.

I used to play on almost every sports team when I was in

middle school. I was the first basewoman, the center, the striker, and the goalie. I also swam competitively on my local swim team, which had practice nearly every day. So when I got sick and had to give up most of these sports, it not only took a toll on my physical health but my mental health as well. I had taken a lot of joy from playing sports, and it was a big part of my life. I used to sleep well at night and be active all day. Now, I couldn't do anything. And, despite being tired, I now realize I had a lot of pent-up mental energy that wasn't getting released by physical exertion.

When I first started practicing yoga, I had heard about some of the health benefits but didn't really think they applied to me. I only picked up a DVD to start practicing because the yogi on the cover was wearing cool clothes. Also, I had tried everything else, so it couldn't hurt.

For the first few weeks that I practiced yoga, I didn't see any noticeable benefits. What I did notice was that, unlike any other physical activities I tried when sick, I didn't feel any worse after doing yoga. That felt like a win. Then I worked with my doctor at the environmental health clinic who told me to (metaphorically) throw away the trendy clothes and practice a therapeutic style of yoga at the clinic. It was when I started practicing this therapeutic version of yoga that I noticed I felt relaxed and had more energy after class—and slept better at night.

I even tried restorative yoga classes which, at first, I wasn't interested in, as I could lie around on pillows at home, thank you very much. But after trying a few of the classes, I realised that yoga didn't need to be fast-moving. Yoga could be active resting with an experienced guide there to help me find a place of balance.

Varying my yoga practice with different styles helped me address the different things I was struggling with. One practice might help me build strength, one relieve tension, and another get a deep session of rest.

A good yoga practice is about finding balance. Balance between effort and relaxation, between strength and flexibility, by listening to your body and meeting yourself where you are on the mat each day. Yoga doesn't care about what you did yesterday or last week or last year; each yoga practice is a new beginning where you can nourish your body in the way that it needs right now.

Evening routines

When working with insomnia, the first yoga practice I recommend adding to your day is an evening routine. The routines I include in this chapter are designed to lower your stress levels and activate the parasympathetic nervous system. I'm incorporating two routines for evening practice. One is a restorative yoga routine that I like to think of as active resting. The other is a combination of the hatha and yin styles. It's more energetic than the restorative practice but still designed to help you get to sleep at night. These routines can be practiced from any time after dinner to just before bed.

What you'll need:

- Yoga mat
- Two to three firm yoga bolsters, pillows, or cushions
- Two blankets
- A yoga strap, scarf, or belt
- Two yoga blocks, hardcover books, or another alternative

Evening Routine 1: Restorative

Supported Reclining Bound Angle Pose

Make a T shape with your blocks and lay one or two long pillows on top of them to create a place for you to recline. Lie back on the recliner; if your neck feels strained, fold a pillow under your head for support. Bring the soles of your feet together and roll two more blankets to place under your thighs. If the blankets are not high enough for you, use pillows or cushions instead. The goal is not for your knees to get to the floor, but for us to bring the floor up to your knees, so don't be afraid to use a lot of props here!

Hold for three to five minutes.

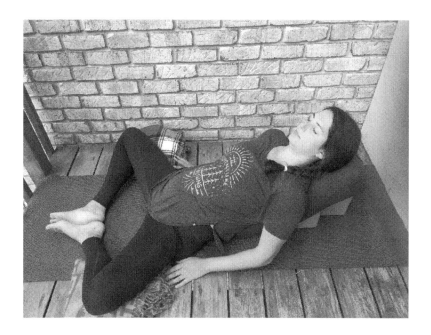

Supported Twists

Lay your pillow or bolster lengthwise along the mat. Bring your right hip to the end of the bolster and lay down, resting your belly on the pillow and your hands on the floor on either side. Rest your left ear on the pillow and look to the right.

Hold for three to five minutes and then switch sides.

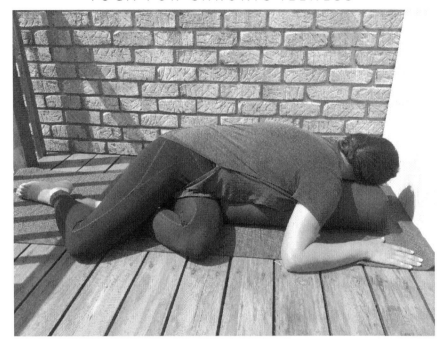

Supported Child's Pose

Create a T shape with the blocks in the middle of your mat and lay one to two pillows on top. Bring your feet together and sit back on your heels, spreading your knees out to either side of the pillows. Walk your hands forward so that your chest rests on the pillows, and rest your right ear on the pillow. If you need more height, fold a blanket under your head. If it's sore on your knees or ankles, roll a blanket to place behind the knees, or fold a blanket to kneel on. If your hips are hanging, you may find it comfortable to place a third pillow under your hips.

Hold for three minutes, switch your head to the opposite side, and hold for another three minutes.

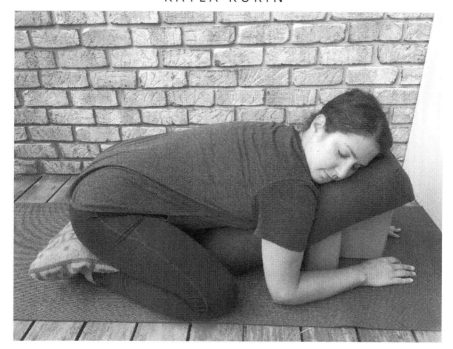

Supported Side Bend

Lay one of the pillows widthwise across the mat. Bring your left hip against the side of the pillow and lay over top of it, perhaps resting your head on your left arm. You can reach your right arm overhead or leave it by your side, whichever is more comfortable for you!

Hold for three to five minutes.

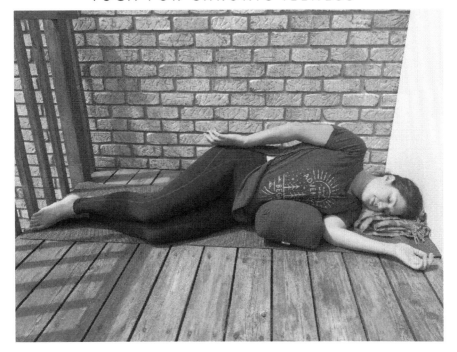

Legs Up the Wall Pose

   Place a pillow and folded blanket against the wall and fold a blanket for under your head. Sit perpendicular to the cushion, lean back, and swing your legs up onto the wall. Adjust the blanket for your head as needed. If the stretch is too intense in the hamstrings, move the pillow a few inches away from the wall to reduce the angle on your legs.

   Hold for five minutes.

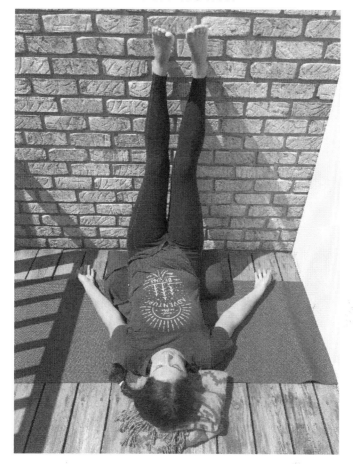

Supported Savasana

Place one or two pillows widthwise across the lower end of your mat and fold a blanket for under your head. Lay down on the mat, bringing the pillows under your knees. Allow your feet to splay open and let your arms rest by your side.

Hold for five to ten minutes. Feel free to add in a meditation or pranayama exercise to this pose.

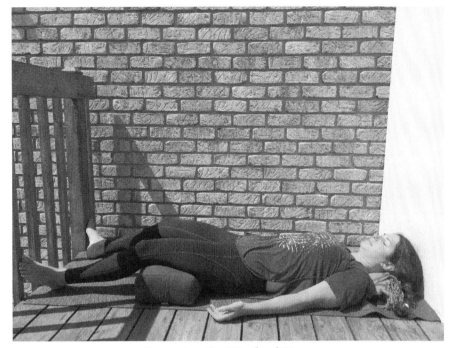

Routine 2: Hatha/Yin

Downward-Facing Dog

Start on your hands and knees with your hands under your shoulders and knees under your hips. Press through the hands and feet to lift the knees, send the hips skyward, and press into a downward-facing dog.

1a) Start on your hands and knees, with a pillow in between your arms. As you press up into downward dog, let your head rest on the pillow.

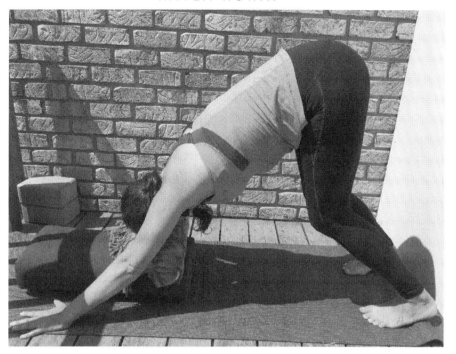

1b) Start on your hands and knees with blocks or books in front of each hand. Bring your hands onto the blocks to press up into downward-facing dog.

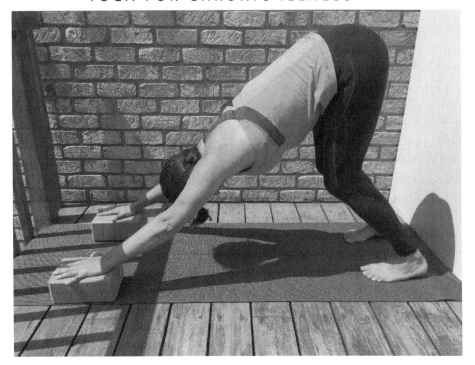

Hold for five to ten breaths.

Seated Twists

Sit in a cross-legged position, perhaps on a pillow or block. Bring the left hand to the right knee and place the right hand behind your hips. Look over your right shoulder. On each inhale, lengthen the spine; on each exhale, twist deeper.

Hold for five to ten breaths and then switch sides.

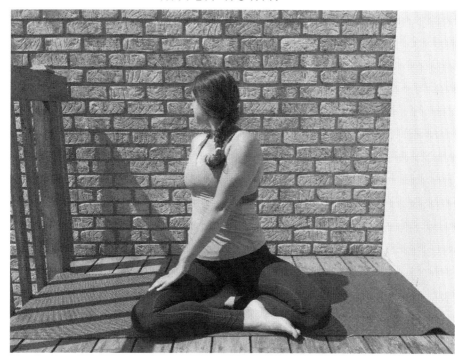

Shoelace Forward Bend

Bring your left foot to your right hip and stack your right leg on top so that from the front it looks almost like a shoelace. Sit up tall and stay here if you feel a stretch in one or both of your hips. If you'd like to go deeper, start to walk your hands forward until you feel a gentle stretch.

If this is too intense, stay in a cross-legged position and walk the hands forward until you feel a stretch in your hips.

Hold for three minutes on each side.

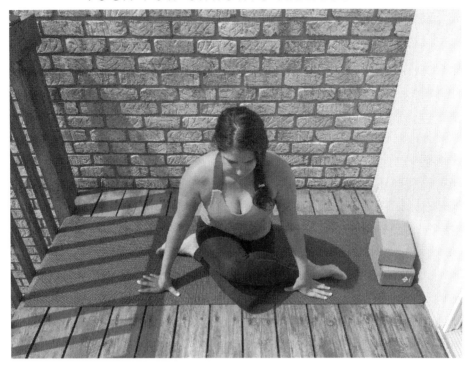

Passive Forward Bend

Place one of the blocks against the wall and stack a pillow lengthwise on top of it (note, if your pillow is not very firm, use the option below), then place a folded blanket on top of the pillow. Sit in a cross-legged position on the floor and lean forward until your forehead rests on the blanket.

4a) Place a folded blanket or pillow on a chair. Sit in a cross-legged position in front of the chair and fold forward until your forehead rests on the chair.

Hold for five minutes.

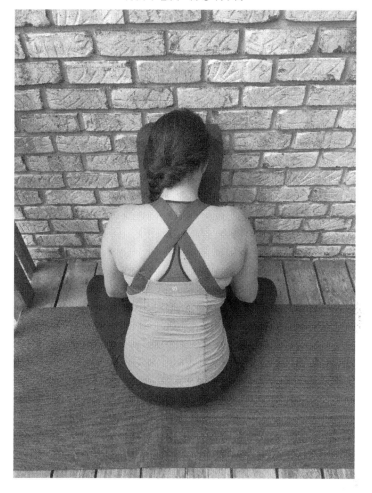

Shoulder Stand

This is one of the more complicated poses in this book. Please look at each step carefully and allow your body to guide you as your best teacher. Do not push further than you need to go. Practicing legs up the wall pose from the first evening routine is an excellent alternative to this pose.

1) Lay down on your mat, placing a folded blanket under your shoulders. Roll your body back as if you are going to do a backward somersault, bending your knees beside your ears and bringing your hands to your lower back for support.

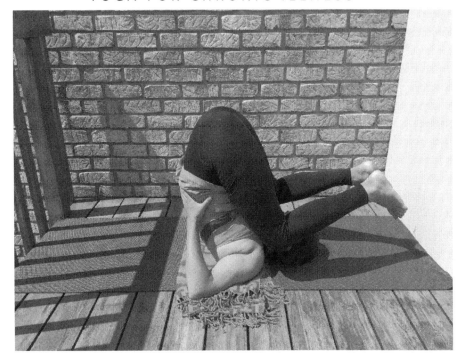

2) If you feel comfortable in this position and want to go further, begin to straighten your legs one at a time toward the ceiling. Continue to support your lower back with your hands and gaze straight ahead. Do not twist your neck from side to side as this can put a strain on your neck muscles.

Stay here for five to ten breaths.

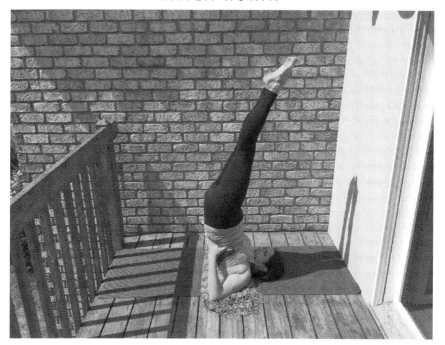

3) To begin our descent, roll both legs behind your head, reaching your toes toward the floor.

Hold for five breaths.

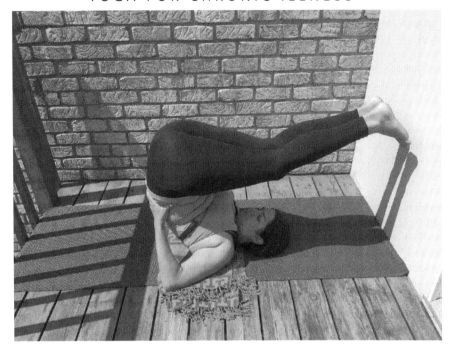

4) Still supporting your back, start to lower your legs slowly and with control back onto the mat.

Supported Backbend

Place one of the pillows widthwise across the top of the mat. Lean back so that the pillow hits between your shoulder blades. If this is uncomfortable for your neck, roll a blanket to place under your neck or head. If the bend is too intense, use a folded blanket rather than pillow under your shoulders.

Hold for one to two minutes.

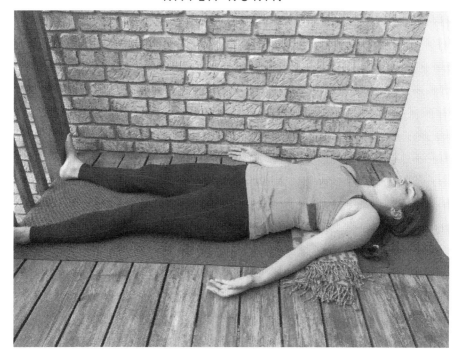

Supported Resting Pose

Make a T with your blocks and lay the pillow over them. Recline on the pillow and use a blanket under your head if needed. Plant your feet on the mat and let your knees fall together.

Hold for five to ten minutes. Feel free to add in a meditation or pranayama exercise to this pose.

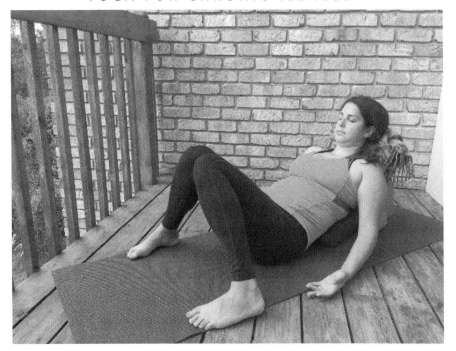

Morning routine

This routine is more energetic than the evening sequences. I recommend doing this in the morning or early afternoon. More rigorous forms of exercise should be avoided in the evening or closer to bed as they can disrupt your sleep schedule.

Child's Pose

With your knees together, sit back on your heels and rest your forehead down on the mat. Get as comfortable as you can in this pose, perhaps placing a blanket or pillow under your head, hips, or ankles.

Hold for ten breaths.

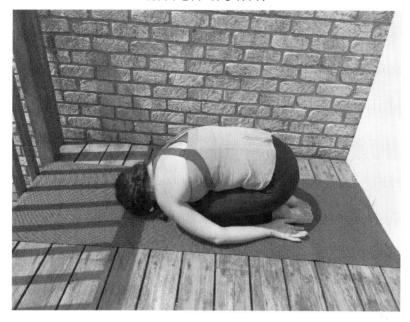

Child's Pose Flow

On your next inhale, "stand up" on your knees and sweep your arms up toward the ceiling. As you exhale, slowly lower back down, resting your forehead on the mat.

Repeat five times.

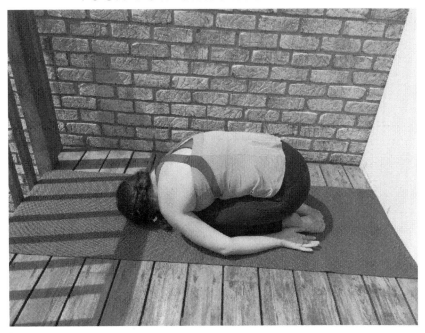

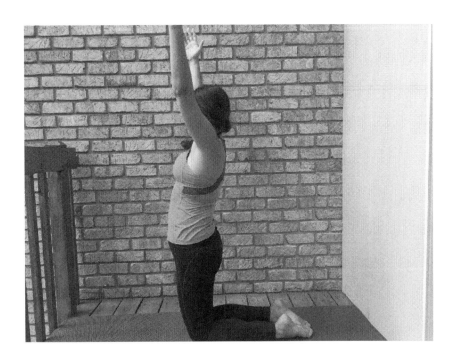

Downward-Facing Dog

Start on your hands and knees with your hands under your shoulders and knees under your hips. Press through the hands and feet to lift the knees, send the hips skyward, and press into a downward-facing dog.

Hold for five to ten breaths.

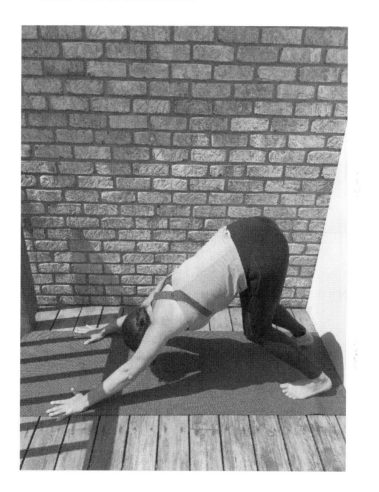

Tadasana

Walk your hands toward your heels, swaying briefly in a forward bend. Bring your hands to your hips and slowly roll up to a standing position. Stand with your feet hip width apart, pressing your toes and heels into the mat. Roll your thighs inward, engage your core muscles (the ones right under your belly button!), and roll your shoulders back. Reach up with your head and neck as if you are a marionette and there is a string attached to the top of your head. Stand up tall, rooting into the ground, feeling your energy building for the day.

Hold for five to ten breaths.

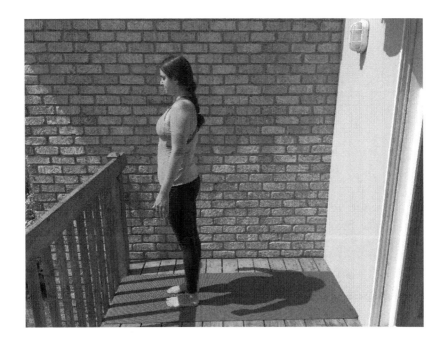

Warrior 1 Flows

From tadasana, sit into a chair pose, sinking the hips down and back so that you can still see your toes, and raise your arms. Then step back with your left foot, planting it on a forty-five-degree angle. Place your hands on your hips to square them to the front, and then extend your arms back up. Hold for five breaths. Step the left foot forward again, straighten the legs, and lower the arms.

Repeat twice on each side.

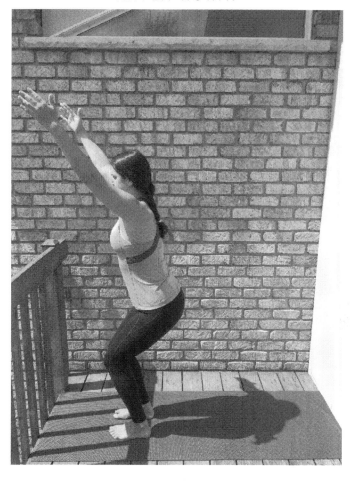

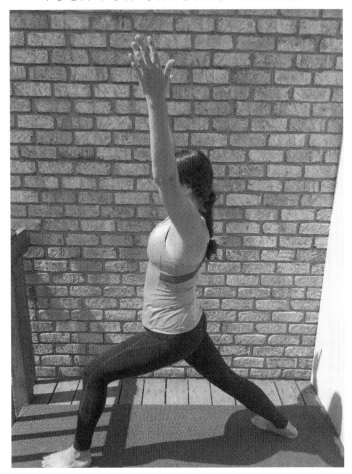

Camel Pose

From standing, lower down onto your knees so that you are "standing" on your knees. Bring both hands to your lower back for support with the fingers facing down. Squeeze the elbows together, push your chest forward, and then from the chest and upper back, begin to bend backward. If it feels good, you can drop your neck behind you, or keep your chin tucked.

Hold for five breaths.

To come out of the pose, reverse the way you came in, first lifting the head and then straightening the spine.

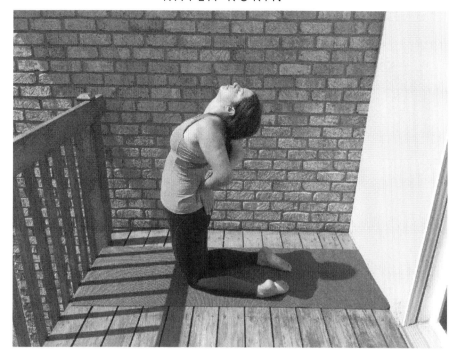

Boat Pose

Sit on the mat with your knees bent and feet planted on the ground. Placing your hands behind you, lift both feet off the ground so that your calves are parallel to the ground.

7a) Bring your hands behind your knees.

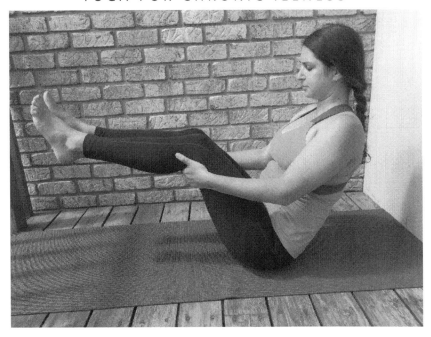

7b) Stretch your arms out beside you, reaching through the fingertips.

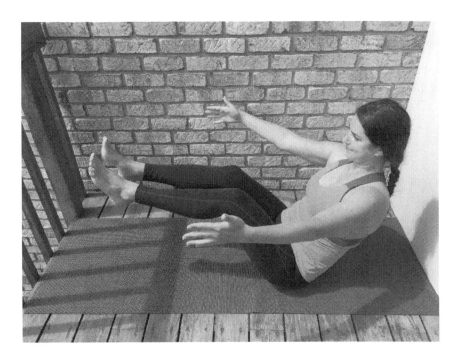

Hold for five breaths.

Sphinx

Lie flat on your stomach. When you're ready to come into the pose, slide your forearms up so that your elbows are under your shoulders. Gaze straight ahead. If this is pinching the lower back, slide your elbows forward until the posture is comfortable.

Hold for ten breaths.

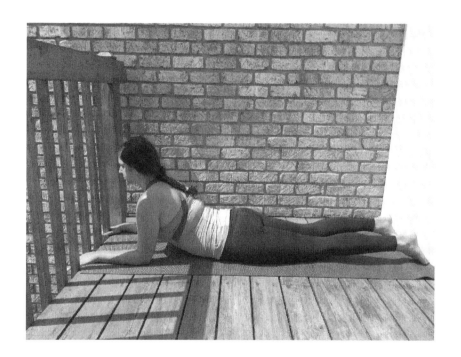

Banasana

Lying on your back, reach your arms overhead and hold your right wrist with your left hand. Reach both arms over to the right. Then shift both legs over to the right, making a "banana" shape.

Hold for two to three minutes on each side.

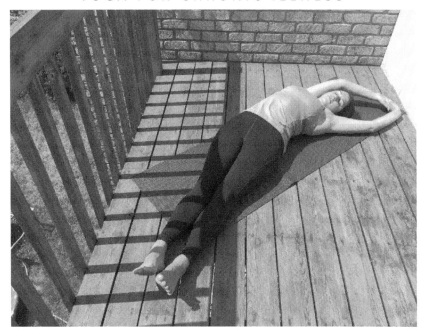

Savasana

Lie comfortably on the mat with your arms by your side and palms facing up. Let your legs and feet fall out to either side. Feel free to use the props from the evening practice in this pose and to add in any of the meditation or pranayama exercises from earlier in the book.

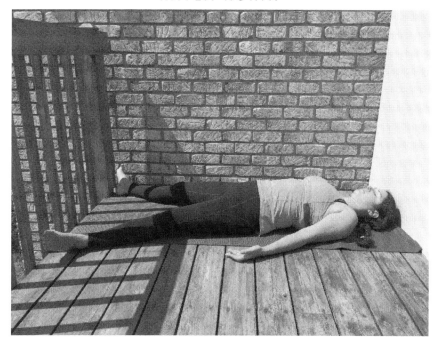

If you'd like to get more morning and evening routines to help with sleep, as well as try some of the breathing exercises and a yoga Nidra practice, check out my ten-day bundle (www.arogayoga.com/online-courses), which includes ten different ten-minute yoga videos for sleep!

What to look for in a yoga class

Yoga is a great therapeutic tool because there need not be any financial or location barriers to your practice. You can use books like this one, YouTube channels, or online providers like Yoga International or Audible Yoga to create a home yoga practice. However, whether you choose to practice at home or with a teacher or therapist, it's still important to find the right teacher and the right style for you.

I hope that you will enjoy the routines I've given in this book as well as the other yogic tips I'm sharing for sleep.

However, you may wish to work with another teacher as well, and that is perfectly fine! Yoga and your journey to wellness are very personal, and if the only thing I give you is help to find the right teacher for you, I will consider this book a success! It can also be beneficial to work with multiple teachers at once or in succession. You don't want to overdo it by practicing too much yoga, but working with teachers with different backgrounds and different perspectives can give you a holistic approach to yoga.

Tips for finding a yoga teacher and classes in your neighbourhood

1. Find a teacher experienced in working with insomnia. Look for a teacher who has lived with insomnia herself or who is an experienced yoga therapist. As with a search for any other type of therapist, you may need to try out a few different teachers until you find the right fit.

2. Look for classes without names like "power" or "intense." These classes tend to focus on aerobic and strength-building exercises rather than on helping the body relax and heal. Look for classes that have the word "gentle" in front of them instead.

3. Notice how you feel in the class. When you do choose a class, make sure you pay attention to how you are feeling during the class. Does the studio feel like a safe and supportive environment? Is the level of intensity in the class appropriate for you? Does the teacher make adaptations for different abilities? These inquiries can all help you determine if you've found the right class or if you need to keep searching.

Styles of yoga to consider

Now let's take a closer look at some of the best styles of yoga for insomnia. Try a few of them out, listen to your body during and after each class, and continue the practice that feels right for you.

Yoga Therapy

Yoga therapy is "the application of yogic principles to a particular person to achieve a particular spiritual, psychological, or physiological goal".[xlv]

Yoga therapy isn't limited to a single style of yoga, and it often includes a combination of different yoga styles, breathwork, meditation, and lifestyle practices. It goes beyond the physical poses, or asanas, of yoga practice, providing a holistic approach to wellness. Yoga therapy is also highly individual. The teacher will ask a lot of questions about your lifestyle and activity levels to help build a practice that is appropriate for you.

Hatha Yoga

Hatha means "force" and is the general term for any type of physical yoga (which applies to most classes we have in the West). But despite the fact that "hatha yoga" can technically refer to any physical yoga practice, you'll find that most classes called hatha are gentle practices that combine basic asanas and breathwork. They're usually less energetic than, for example, vinyasa flow or Ashtanga classes. This is a good option for moderately active people.

Restorative Yoga

This style of yoga is perfect for anyone who needs a deep relaxation. In most therapeutic classes, all of the poses will be practiced either seated or lying down, and the class will move at a slow pace. You'll be led through a series of postures, using props to help make the poses comfortable. Postures are held for several minutes, and the focus is on deep breathing and relaxation.

Yin Yoga

Yin yoga targets the connective tissues and joints of the body. Normally, when we practice yoga, we are working with our muscles and may neglect the deeper tissues in our body. Each pose is held for three to five minutes, and for this reason, students often find that the class is more challenging mentally than physically.

Like any new activity, you should check with your doctor (and listen to your body) when it comes to trying yin yoga. People with hypermobility disorders such as Ehlers-Danlos syndrome should check with their doctors before trying this style and, if given the go-ahead, should make sure to find an experienced teacher to guide them.

Yoga Nidra

If you are unsure of your energy levels and don't yet feel comfortable with physical yoga, this is a great practice to try! Also known as yogic sleep, yoga Nidra is a guided meditation that helps you decrease stress and anxiety. It's a wonderful alternative for people who have tried mindfulness meditation but found they were not able to sink deeply into the practice because their mind was always racing. Because yoga Nidra is guided with words and imagery, many students find it easier to focus and relax during the practice.

Iyengar

"The practice of precision" was created by B.K.S Iyengar. This practice makes use of traditional hatha postures, with an intense focus on alignment. Iyengar practitioners use many props, making it possible for people of many abilities to participate. This style of yoga is trendy among yoga therapists due to its focus on personal adaptations for different bodies.

Restorative Flow Yoga

Restorative flow (also known as slow flow or gentle flow yoga) classes link the breath and movement for a dynamic class. These classes are for people with moderate levels of energy. It is an adaptation of the more energetic vinyasa flow classes that has a more gentle approach.

Final Tips

A private class with the right teacher is a great way to get started. In a private session, the teacher will be able to adapt the sequence to your needs, so you'll have adjustments ready when you attend a group class. If there are no appropriate yoga teachers in your area, look for teachers who can offer classes via Skype or video conferencing. If you're interested in booking a private session with me, you can learn more here (www.arogayoga.com/online-courses). If I don't think it's a good fit, I'm happy to refer you to another teacher.

Lastly, before beginning a yoga practice, you should speak to your doctor to see if it is right for you. Given your medical condition(s), ask if there are any postures you should avoid. If so, make a note of them and inform your teacher so that you can adapt the class together if needed.

Action steps

1) Add yoga goals to your mindful goal setting page.

2) Decide how many times a week you can commit to a short yoga practice.

3) Do it! Roll out your mat, follow the instructions in this book or in the ten-day bundle, and experience the benefits of yoga firsthand!

Step 7: Building a Lifestyle for Better Sleep

People often ask me what the one most beneficial thing I did to overcome insomnia is. I understand why I get asked this question. When I was sick, I wanted to know what change to make or what treatment to focus on that would make a difference or provide a cure. However, the body doesn't work in isolation. There were many different things I tried, and while some did nothing, others contributed to my overall improvement in health, which led to better sleep.

To illustrate how sometimes it can be hard to pinpoint what helped, I'll tell the story of my trip to Maine in university. It was at a time when my roommates and I were all stressed out. It was exam time. My roommates were in their final year of study and worried about their exam results. I was in the lowest depths of illness. I was barely making it to class or getting out of bed, and I had to postpone my exams until later in the semester. So when one of my roommates invited us to visit her family in northern Maine for the weekend, I at first said no. Even though I had never been to Maine and wanted to explore this side of the continent, I felt like I had to stay home and try to study or catch up on my schoolwork, or even just stay in bed and rest. Somehow, my friends convinced me to come with them, and we drove through the snow-covered forests watching the moose prints pass us by on the side of the road.

We stayed with my friend's parents, who had a lovely New England home, two dogs, a cozy lounge with a fireplace, and enough bedrooms for each of us to sleep on our own. When I looked outside my window, all I could see was snow and trees. We went to the mall and got mani-pedis (something I had never done spontaneously before), went shopping, ate lobster chowder, and didn't think at all about school.

When I returned to Halifax, I was able to get more of my work done and concentrate more on studying than I had been able to before. Was it Maine that was the magic pill? Was it nature? Spending time with friends? Getting my ears pierced or a mani-pedi? Was it the mindfulness that I find often accompanies travel? Did I need more lobster in my life?

The truth is, it wasn't one of those things; it was all of those things. It was how each of those actions helped me reduce some of the stress I was feeling, eat healthy (read: non-student) food, and have fun.

It took me a few more years until I was able to apply this principle to my life entirely. It wasn't just doing yoga or eating well or traveling that would help me feel better. It was creating a lifestyle that was nourishing in a variety of ways, as well as addressing specific health problems, that helped me feel better, sleep better, and live better.

In the following pages are some of what has contributed to

my improved sleep and healthier lifestyle.

Massage

Working with an experienced massage therapist can help you relieve both muscular and psychological stress and tension.

If you often wake up sore and stiff and have a lot of muscular tension when trying to fall asleep, a deep tissue massage may help you get rid of some of that tension and sleep better.

If a more significant challenge for you is a racing mind, an Ayurvedic head massage or full-body oil massage can relieve mental stress.

Most of us can't afford to get a professional massage on a daily or weekly basis, so starting a self-massage routine in the evening can be an enjoyable way to relax before bed.

The first step to starting your massage is choosing the massage oil. If you have dry skin, use a heavy oil such as sesame, almond, or avocado. For sensitive skin or skin that's often red, use a cooling or neutral oil such as olive, coconut, or castor oil. For oily skin, use a light oil such as flaxseed.

Once you have your oil ready, you can heat it over the stove or use it at room temperature. Begin with your legs and work your way up your body to your head. There are many different techniques to use for massage. I usually start with a warming rub of the area, then search out areas of tension to apply pressure. Hold areas of tension for five to ten seconds, and then massage around the area. It's hard to injure yourself or do harm with a self-massage, so really anything that feels good to you can help relieve stress and pain.

If you do see a massage therapist semiregularly, you can ask for help creating a daily self-massage routine for in between professional massages.

Going to visit a masseuse often also means a visit to an

oasis of calm, whether it's in a spa or massage parlor, and continuing this ritual at home can help create a calming evening routine for you.

Spa

Since the ancient Greeks, humans have been using water treatments to improve health. Before around 400 BCE, bathing was mostly for cleansing purposes. However, the doctor Hippocrates (from the Hippocratic oath) believed that many diseases centered around an imbalance of bodily fluids.

The Greeks weren't the only ones with this idea. You may be familiar with the Japanese Onsen, Turkish hammams, or Finnish saunas—all water- or steam-based spa treatments originating in different parts of the world.

Visiting a spa can literally wash away your stress. Increasing body temperature can help soothe muscles and joints. Also, the relaxing nature of spas can help activate your parasympathetic nervous system, creating a space of healing for you.

It's also a great way to start building joy into your self-care. Going to the spa is fun, and an activity you can do with friends and family. Bringing joy, fun, and community into your spa experience will only increase the healing benefits.

Going in the evening or later in the afternoon can help begin relaxing your body and mind for sleep.

Exercise

Yoga isn't the only form of exercise that's beneficial to insomnia. Exercise is good for your health, period.

Exercising, especially earlier in the day, has been proven to help with sleep (in addition to a host of other health concerns like weight loss, mood, anxiety, and more).

I encourage you to experiment with any exercise you like, whether it's soccer, dance, running, *etc.* Start slow and do each exercise mindfully, listening if your body tells you to stop.

The best routine is the one that you can stick with, but if you can add cardiovascular or strength exercise to your weekly routine in addition to yoga, the benefits will be exponential.

Food

"Eat food, not too much, mostly plants." – Michael Pollan

I'm always hesitant to give dietary advice in my writing because trying different extreme diets has become trendy, which makes figuring out what to eat overwhelming. Not to mention the shame-based way we think about food and weight in modern society.

However, I do think food can be a massive tool in improving your health. I do not think anyone should feel bad about their weight, severely restrict their eating, or try a new crash or fad diet to try to "cleanse" or "lose weight." One great thing that's come out of my healing journey is that I appreciate my body for what it can do, not for how it looks.

Food can be a tool for helping your body heal and feel its best. It can also affect sleep either by promoting sleep or by impeding your body's ability to create the right sleep secretions.

Sleep-specific food recommendations:
These substances have been shown to disrupt sleep. If you must ingest them, do so before noon.
- Caffeine (coffee, tea, chocolate, and more)
- Alcohol
- Marijuana[4]

- Nicotine
- Sugar (fruit sugar is okay, but avoid after dinner)

These foods may help promote sleep and should be consumed in the evening.

- For dinner, eat a warm meal (perhaps soup or curry) and avoid cold, raw foods like salad or sushi
- Chamomile tea
- Valerian root tea
- Warm dairy (if not lactose intolerant); this might include heated milk, a cream sauce, or melted cheese
- Meat, especially turkey, contains tryptophan which, if you choose to consume meat, can help you sleep better

Ayurvedic food recommendations:

Vata is related to the element of air. When Vata is in excess, this can lead to symptoms such as bloating, gassiness, diarrhea, and constipation. To combat these effects, Ayurveda recommends consuming warm and nourishing foods and staying away from raw foods like smoothies and salads. Stick to warm soups, curries, rice dishes, and cooked vegetables.

Healthy fats and oils are recommended for decreasing Vata dosha, and even a sweetener such as honey can be used in a hot ginger tea. Rice and wheat are considered the best grains for Vata imbalance, while the best fruits are those that are denser, such as bananas, avocados, mangoes, berries, and figs. Minimize bean consumption, as beans can cause gas. But cheese lovers can rejoice, because dairy is recommended for balancing Vata!

---

4. While you're unlikely to consume alcohol or marijuana in the morning, limiting its usage to early evening or a small dosage can help support better sleep.

General food recommendations:

Despite the many fad diets out there, research still shows that the most effective diet we have in terms of improving our health and preventing disease is a plant-based one. If you can cut down on meat products and focus on including fresh vegetables, fruits, legumes, and whole grains into your diet, you should see a positive difference. For sleep, cutting down on caffeinated and sugary foods and drinks at all times, but especially in the afternoon or evening, will make it easier for your brain to create the hormones that promote sleep.

Cutting down on processed foods and sticking to fresh produce (fruits, vegetables, fresh meat and fish, grains like rice, oats, quinoa, *etc.*) is the simplest way to improve your diet.

Dharma

Dharma is a Sanskrit word that doesn't have a direct English translation but is often used to signify doing your life's work. It may feel out of place talking about your life's purpose in a book on yoga for insomnia. But I think that finding what you are supposed to do in life can have a significant impact on your life, health, and stress levels and can be directly related to sleep.

When you're not doing the thing that feels joyous and meaningful to you, life can feel pointless or unsatisfactory. It can be challenging to make decisions that are good for your health when you do not feel like you are fulfilled in life. Many people (and I have been here) turn to booze, smoking, drugs, food, or sex as a way to fill the void of something that is missing in their lives, or perhaps just from boredom.

One challenge with finding your dharma is that, if you are imbalanced, it can be hard to know what it is that you want or what will bring meaning to your life. When you're in a state of Ayurvedic imbalance, it's believed you will make decisions to increase this imbalance. If you are moving toward balancing your doshas, you will begin to make decisions that continue bringing you toward balance.

If you are feeling lost and like you don't know what your life's purpose is—or perhaps you thought you knew until you became ill—practicing yoga and meditation can help lead you toward finding or rediscovering your dharma.

When you are living the life you are truly meant to live, you will find it easier to make healthy choices. You may find yourself feeling less restless and less stressed when you get into bed after spending a day doing what you love.

I can't tell you what your dharma is, but if you follow the yoga and meditation practices in this book and make a habit of listening to and acting upon the things your body and your mind are telling you, you will be well on your way to finding the thing it is you need to be doing in this world.

Your dharma may be a career, taking care of people, creating art, or some combination of these things and more. Feeling as though you are living a life of purpose can add years to your life.

Action steps

1) Write down any activities from this chapter you'd like to try to improve your sleep and add them to your yogic goal chart.
2) Schedule in time for these activities.
3) Decide whether you'd like to make changes to your diet. If so, create a meal plan and grocery list.
4) Think about if you are living your life's purpose, and if not, could that be obstructing your sleep and causing you other health problems? Perhaps explore this issue with a partner, close friend, or therapist.

Final Thoughts

At the height of my struggle with insomnia and chronic fatigue, I often got asked how I was doing. Did I feel tired? How tired? What did the tired feel like? Did I feel sleepy at night? Was my mind racing? Was my leg shaking? Did I have trouble relaxing?

No doctor ever asked me questions beyond my symptoms, like what helped me feel relaxed, what made me feel energized, what made me forget about my stresses and worries. I was in a world of reactionary medicine. Doctors wanted to find a solution to the problem that was occurring, not ask why the problem had started in the first place. They wanted to be able to prescribe me a medication or some other treatment, rather than find the things I was already doing that helped me to feel energized during the day, relaxed in the evening, and less stressed overall.

I often felt like I had to cut out things that made me feel better to get my health back. Things like a later bedtime and wake up time (full night owl here), going out with friends in the evening, and foods I enjoyed. In part, I did. I needed to set boundaries, and I needed to play the role of detective to find out which factors were affecting my sleep and which were not. I think this is the way with all chronic health conditions that have no known cure. One needs to use the power of deduction to find strategies that work for you as an individual. Yet we need to be asking the right questions and acknowledging the roles that stress and happiness play in our overall health.

If I didn't have to feel guilty for continuing to play a couple of sports because I didn't have the energy to do schoolwork— would I have spent less time tossing and turning at night? If I was allowed to plan my year abroad with abandon rather than wondering if my health would be good enough and if this was too self-indulgent—would my health have improved due to lack of worry?

Sleeping is essential to our ability to heal, enjoy more energy during the day, and maintain a positive mood. Yet no one was looking at the other pillars of my life to help me with sleep. What was causing the stress that was keeping me up at night?

I hope that the tips and tools I've provided in this book help you assess your sleep and your sleep patterns. I also hope that instead of feeling like you now have to be restricted in what you're able to do, you feel that you have more power to choose. To choose the things that make you feel good, to choose to drink hot chocolate at night now and then if it makes you feel happy, and to decide to cancel plans with a friend if you know you don't have the energy to go out right now. Choosing to live mindfully, right at this moment, and able to make the myriad of small choices that help you sleep better.

As I got older, I was finally able to start addressing the root causes of my stress. While it can sometimes be hard to transport back into the mind of teenage me, I can observe myself now, on nights when I find myself tossing and turning for longer than usual. Did I miss a yoga practice? Am I unhappy in my work? Life? Am I feeling stress from an unknown cause? Why might these patterns be presenting themselves? Understanding the underlying concepts of sleep and what kept me up at night helps me now identify the causes of an occasional restless night.

This is something that even the most perfect sleep medication could not have given me: the ability to understand myself and thus help myself find the best night's sleep that I can.

I hope that the tools that worked for me also help you in some way and that you can find a better night's sleep and lead a more balanced life.

Sleep well.

Thank You!

I hope you've enjoyed this book and you now have some concrete ideas on how yoga can help you recover from insomnia. If you enjoyed this book, I would love it if you could leave a review on Amazon or Goodreads. Your honest review will help me get this information out to more people living with insomnia! If you have any questions about anything in this book or would like to update me on your progress, I'd love to hear from you at kayla@arogayoga.com!

About the Author

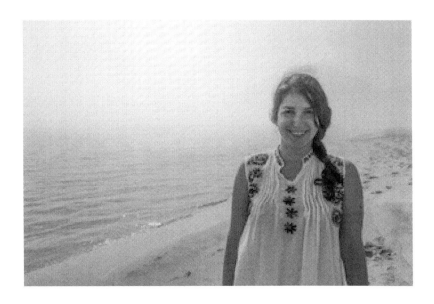

Kayla Kurin is the author of <u>Yoga for Chronic Fatigue</u>, <u>Yoga for Chronic Pain</u>, and Yoga for Insomnia. She is a yoga therapist, writer, and constant traveler who is always ready to embark on her next adventure and share what she's learned with humor, compassion, and kindness. You can learn more about her on her website: <u>arogayoga.com.</u>

Endnotes

[i] Aaron A. Hanyu-Deutmeyer;Scott C. Dulebohn *Pain, Phantom Limb* (Statpearls: April 17, 2018: https://www.ncbi.nlm.nih.gov/books/NBK448188/)

[ii] . Sympathetic Nervous System Indeed!... And Why Some People Suffer Over Your Pain (Bodyinmind.org August 2017: https://bodyinmind.org/meaning-pain-giummarra/)

iii. Lara Hilton et al. *Mindfulness Meditation for Chronic Pain: Systemic Review and Meta-analysis* (Annals of Behavioral Medicine 2017; 51(2): 199–213: https://www.ncbi.nlm.nih.gov/pmc/articles/PMC5368208/)

iv. Chris C. Streeter at al. *Effects of Yoga Versus Walking on Mood, Anxiety, and Brain GABA levels* (Journal of Alternative and Complementary Medicine 2010 Nov; 16(11): 1145–1152: https://www.ncbi.nlm.nih.gov/pmc/articles/PMC3111147/)

[v] Turan, B., Foltz, C., Cavanagh, J. F., Wallace, B. A., Cullen, M., Rosenberg, E. L., Jennings, P., Ekman, P., & Kemeny, M. E. (2015).Anticipatory Sensitization to Repeated Stressors: the role of initital cortisol reactivity and meditation/emotion skills training. Psychoneuroendocrinology, 52, 229-238

vi. Ankad RD et al. *Effect of short-term Pranayama and Meditation on Cardiovascular Functions in Healthy Individuals* (Heart Views 2011 Apr;12(2):58-62:

https://www.ncbi.nlm.nih.gov/pubmed/22121462)

Matarelli D, Cocchioni M, Scuri S, Pompei P. *Diaphragmatic Breathing Reduce Postprandial Oxidative Stress* (J Altern Complement Med. 2011 Jul;17(7):623-8:

https://www.ncbi.nlm.nih.gov/pubmed/21688985

[vii] Alyson Ross et al. Evid Based Complement Alternat Med. 2012; 2012: 983258.
Published online 2012 Aug 14.doi:10.1155/2012/983258

[viii] Ranganathan VK[1],Siemionow V,Liu JZ,Sahgal V,Yue GH Neuropsychologia.2004;42(7):944-56.

ix. Francon A, Forestier R. *Spa Therapy in Rheumatology* (Bull Acad Natl Med.2009 Jun;193(6):1345-56:

https://www.ncbi.nlm.nih.gov/pubmed/20120164)

[x] Jefferson R Roberts, Chronic Fatigue Syndrome (CFS), https://emedicine.medscape.com/article/235980-overview.
[xi] James P Griffith, Fahd A Zarrouf, A Systemic Review of Chronic Fatigue Syndrome: Don't Assume It's Depression, Prim Care Companion J Clin Psychiatry. 2008; 10(2): 120–128.
[xii] Anthony L. Komaroff. Inflammation correlates with symptoms in chronic fatigue syndrome. PNASAugust 22, 2017114(34)8914-8916;published ahead of print August 15, 2017https://doi.org/10.1073/pnas.1712475114
[xiii] Rimes, K. A., Ashcroft, J., Bryan, L., & Chalder, T. (2016). Emotional suppression in chronic fatigue syndrome: Experimental study.Health Psychology, 35(9), 979-986. http://dx.doi.org/10.1037/hea0000341
[xiv] Kurin, Kayla. Ayurvedic Tips for Chronic Fatigue. Yoga

International: https://yogainternational.com/article/view/ayurvedic-tips-for-chronic-fatigue

[xv] Marshall, Kester. Chronic Fatigue and Fibromyalgia: An Ayurvedic PerspectiveMuditaInstitute: http://www.muditainstitute.com/articles/ayurvedicmedicine/cfs fibromyalgia.html

[xvi] The resilience of the intestinal microbiota influences health and disease Felix Sommer,Jacqueline Moltzau Anderson,Richa Bharti,Jeroen Raes&Philip Rosenstiel. Nature Reviews Microbiologyvolume15,630–638(2017)

[xvii] Torgan, Carol. Placebo effect in depression treatment. National Institutes of Health. October 19, 2015. https://www.nih.gov/news-events/nih-research-matters/placebo-effect-depression-treatment

[xviii] Sollie, K., Næss, E. T., Solhaug, I., &Thimm, J. C. (2017). Mindfulness training for chronic fatigue syndrome: apilot study. Health Psychology Report, 5(3), 240–250. doi: https://doi.org/10.5114/hpr.2017.65469

[xix] Tara Sampalli,Elizabeth Berlasso,Roy Fox,andMark Petter. A controlled study of the effect of a mindfulness-based stress reduction technique in women with multiple chemical sensitivity, chronic fatigue syndrome, and fibromyalgia. J Multidiscip Healthc. 2009; 2: 53–59.

[xxi] Katharine A. RimesJanet Wingrove. Mindfulness-Based Cognitive Therapy for People with Chronic Fatigue Syndrome Still Experiencing Excessive Fatigue after Cognitive Behaviour Therapy: A Pilot Randomized Study. Wiley online library. https://onlinelibrary.wiley.com/doi/abs/10.1002/cpp.793

[xxii]Britta K.HölzelabJamesCarmodycMarkVangelaChristinaCongletonaSita M.YerramsettiaTimGardabSara W.Lazara Mindfulness practice leads to increases in regional brain grey matter

density. Psychiatry Research: Neuroimaging

Volume 191, Issue 1,30 January 2011, Pages 36-43

[xxiii] Oka, Takakazu, et al. Isometric yoga improves the fatigue and pain of patients with chronic fatigue syndrome who are resistant to conventional therapy: a randomized, controlled trial. Biopsychosoc Med. 2014; 8: 27.

[xxiv] Chris C Streeter et al. Effects of Yoga Versus Walking on Mood, Anxiety, and Brain GABA Levels: A Randomized Controlled MRS Study. 8 Nov 2010https://doi.org/10.1089/acm.2010.0007

Satish GurunathraoPatilaShankargouda S.PatilbManjunatha R.AithalaaKusal KantiDasa. Comparison of yoga and walking-exercise on cardiac time intervals as a measure of cardiac function in elderly with increased pulse pressure. Indian Heart JournalVolume 69, Issue 4,July–August 2017, Pages 485-490

xxv. Thomas M. Heffron, "Insomnia Awareness Day Facts and Stats," *Sleep Education*, last modified March 10, 2014, http://sleepeducation.org/news/2014/03/10/insomnia-awareness-day-facts-and-stats.

xxvi. Pete Evans, "More Than A Quarter of Canadians Get Fewer Than 7 Hours of Sleep," *CBC*, last modified March 18, 2017, https://www.cbc.ca/news/business/lack-of-sleep-rand-1.4029406.

xxvii. "Sleep and Sleep Disorders," *Centers for Disease Control and Prevention*, last modified August 8, 2018, **https://www.cdc.gov/sleep/**about_sleep/chronic_disease.html.

xxviii. Robbert Havekes, Alan J. Park, Jennifer C. Tudor,

et al., Sleep deprivation causes memory deficits by negatively impacting neuronal connectivity in hippocampal area CA1. Groningen Institute for Evolutionary Life Sciences (GELIFES), University of Groningen, Groningen 9747 AG, The Netherlands.

xxix. Michelle A. Short and Mia Louca, "Sleep deprivation leads to mood deficits in healthy adolescents," *Sleep Medicine* 16, no. 8 (August 2015): 987-993.

xxx. A. Rechtschaffen, M.A. Gilliland, B.M. Bergmann, and J.B. Winter,

"Physiological correlates of prolonged sleep deprivation in rats," *Science* 221, no. 4606 (July 1983): 182-184.

xxxi. Masayo Kojima, Kenji Wakai, Takashi Kawamura, Akiko Tamakoshi, Rie Aoki, Yingsong Lin, Toshiko Nakayama, Hiroshi Horibe, Nobuo Aoki, and Yoshiyuki Ohno, "Sleep Patterns and Total Mortality: A 12-Year Follow-up Study in Japan Journal of Epidemiology," 2000 年 10 巻 2 号 p. 87-93.

xxxii. Stanley Coren, *Sleep Thieves* (New York: Simon and Schuster, 1996): 30.

xxxiii. J. Seligman, S.S. Felder, and M.E. Robinson, "Substance Abuse and Mental Health Services Administration," *Disaster Med Public Health Prep* (June 2016).

xxxiv. Timothy McCall, *Yoga As Medicine* (New York: Bantam Books, 2007): 413.

xxxv. Jason C. Ong *et al.,* "A Randomized Controlled

Trial of Mindfulness Meditation for Chonric Insomnia: Effects on Daytime Symptoms and Cognitive-Emotional Arousal," *Springer Link* 9, no. 6 (December 2018): 1702-1712.

xxxvi. T. Kamei, Y. Toriumi, H. Kimura, H. Kumano, S. Ohno, and K. Kimura, "Decrease in Serum Cortisol during Yoga Exercise is Correlated with Alpha Wave Activation," *Perceptual and Motor Skills* 90, no. 3 (2000): 1027–1032.

xxxvii. Kasiganesan Harinath, Anand Sawarup Malhotra, Karan Pal, Rajendra Prasad, Rajesh Kumar, Trilok Chand Kain, Lajpat Rai, and Ramesh Chand Sawhney, "Effects of Hatha Yoga and Omkar Meditation on Cardiorespiratory Performance, Psychologic Profile, and Melatonin Secretion," *The Journal of Alternative and Complementary Medicine* 10, no. 2 (July 5, 2004).

xxxviii. Shirley Telles, Shivangi Pathak, Ankur Kumar, Prabhat Mishra, and Acharya Balkrishna A., "Ayurvedic Doshasas Predictors of Sleep Quality," *Med Sci Monit* 21 (2015): 1421–1427.

xxxix. Patrice Voss, Maryse E. Thomas, J. Miguel Cisneros-Franco, and Étienne de Villers-Sidani, "Dynamic Brains and the Changing Rules of Neuroplasticity: Implications for Learning and Recovery,"
Front Psychol 8 (2017).

xl. Madhuri R.A. Tolahunase, Rajesh Sagar, Muneeba Faiq, and Rimaa Dada, "Yoga- and meditation-based lifestyle intervention increases neuroplasticity and reduces severity of major depressive disorder: A randomized controlled trial," *Restorative Neurology and Neuroscience* 36, no. 3 (2018): 423-442.

xli. Sue McGreevey, "Eight weeks to a better brain," *The Harvard Gazette*, last modified January 21, 2011, https://news.harvard.edu/gazette/story/2011/01/eight-weeks-to-a-better-brain/.

xlii. J.A. Horne and A.J. Reid, "Night-time sleep EEG changes following body heating in a warm bath," *Electroencephalography and Clinical Neurophysiology 60, no. 2* (February 1985): 154-157.

xliii. Marie-Pierre St-Onge, PhD; Amy Roberts, PhD; Ari Shechter, PhD; and Arindam Roy Choudhury, PhD. "Fibre and Saturated Fat Are Associated with Sleep Arousals and Slow Wave Sleep," *Journal of Clinical Sleep Medicine* 12 no. 01.

xliv. Stanley Coren, *Sleep Thieves*, 137.

xlv. International Association of Yoga Therapists, https://www.iayt.org/.

Printed in Great Britain
by Amazon